MIGRAINE

UNDERSTANDING AND COPING
WITH MIGRAINE

Ann

Thorsons
An Imprint of HarperCollinsPublishers

Thorsons
An Imprint of HarperCollins*Publishers*
77–85 Fulham Palace Road,
Hammersmith, London W6 8JB
1160 Battery Street
San Francisco, California 94111–1213

Published by Thorsons 1996
1 3 5 7 9 10 8 6 4 2

A catalogue record for this book
is available from the British Library

ISBN 0 7225 3265 2

Printed and bound in Great Britain by
Caledonian International Book Manufacturing Ltd, Glasgow

CONTENTS

Not only what you eat but when you eat it – the role of low blood sugar .
Dieting and migraine . Alcohol and caffeine . The importance of a good
diet . Sleep . The role of sleep. The stages of sleep . Sleep as a treatment .
The menstrual cycle . The role of hormones . Other cyclical phenomena.

headache history . The questions your doctor will ask you . Questions you should ask your doctor . Misunderstandings that can arise . Points of friction . When your doctor will refer you to a specialist . A clean sheet . Your rights . What to do if you cannot get on with your doctor . Clinics — where, when and how . When do you need a clinic? . What are the advantages of a clinic? . What are the disadvantages? . Where to go . How to prepare — what to expect . The follow-up . Clinical research . Who else can help? . Self-help groups . Organizations that give help . The role of those closest to you .

7   The Way Ahead   140

Current research . What is being done? . The international scene . Scientific and clinical research . Taking part in research . Quality of life . The impact of migraine . Factors affecting perception . The belittling of migraine . The way ahead . No need to apologize . Raising awareness . There is always something you can do . Taking it a day at a time . What to aim for — evaluating your progress .

FOREWORD

There are two types of medical charities: those that are doctor-led and those that are patient-led. The Migraine Trust, since its inception in 1965, has belonged to the first group and has trustees and a medical advisory board. Its Director, always a lay person, has to tackle innumerable questions from a host of worried migraine sufferers. The Director thus becomes aware of the problems that patients have and, over the years, becomes expert in finding the answers. These can be given in everyday language, avoiding the technical jargon to which doctors are prone. It is this ability to communicate in a way patients can understand that gives this book the edge over books for migraine sufferers written by medical experts.

Since its foundation over 30 years ago, the Migraine Trust has had five directors, but Ann Rush is the first to have had the courage and persistence to write a book. It is particularly important at this time, when health service provision throughout the world is coming under close inspection because of financial considerations.

Inevitably those disorders that are considered not to be serious – that is, fatal – receive less attention and less sympathy than they deserve. It is particularly in these areas that charities such as the Migraine Trust find their complementary niche, filling a serious gap in health provision and, indeed, providing funds for much-needed migraine clinics and important research.

All seven chapters in this book make the many problems of migraine understandable. The initial overview tells us about its history and possible causes. The second chapter describes the different types of attacks and how they vary throughout life, while the third chapter classifies the different types of migraine and other types of headache. The next chapter on management will be of particular interest to sufferers, not least because it will help them to study their own lifestyle and, by its modification, prevent attacks, so avoiding drug therapy. Inevitably there will be some patients who will need drug treatment, though, and the fifth chapter will help in understanding the various side-effects that arise. Chapter 6, on how to get help, will also prove of value to those who have had problems in getting good advice, whilst the final chapter gives hope for the future. There are also very useful appendices – a reading list, useful addresses, index and further reference.

This book is ideal for patients with migraine and, indeed, there will be few doctors who would not learn a great deal from its contents. It is unique in its fresh and clear approach and Ann Rush is to be congratulated on a magnificent effort. It will undoubtedly help the many hundreds of thousands of migraine sufferers, each of whom will find answers within its covers.

Dr F. Clifford Rose, FRCP, London Neurological Centre

1

AN OVERVIEW

Where to start

Every person is individual and, with a condition as complicated and varied as migraine, this means that every attack is individual, too. Migraine sufferers seem to have an inbuilt sensitivity or vulnerability to various stimuli that is probably inherited. These may be triggers from the outside world, such as food or climate, or vulnerabilities from within, such as a sensitivity to changes in hormonal levels. Their bodies seem unable to cope with what, for others, are normal processes the body carries out automatically. Even pleasurable things – like eating a good meal, listening to music, relaxing in front of the television, snuggling down for a lie-in at the weekend, watching sunlight on snow, going on holiday – can cause a migraine to strike in such a person .

Some think of migraine as an inbuilt sensitivity to just living. It is a blow to the system that reverberates throughout the body. During an attack they are themselves, but not quite themselves, subtly different, a distortion of their real selves.

BEING HONEST WITH YOURSELF –
DEFINING THE PROBLEMS

Whether you have just been diagnosed as having migraine or you have been suffering for years, start reading as if you were a complete beginner. This book will help to answer your questions and provide the information that will enable you to understand and successfully manage your attacks.

I have talked to many migraine sufferers during the years I have been at The Migraine Trust, one of the world's leading research charities into migraine. Not only do we fund research and hold international symposia and workshops for researchers, but we have also developed a wide-ranging service for sufferers as we are only too aware of the urgent need to give help and information and answer the questions of sufferers who are often desperate to find answers. All kinds of people turn to us; perhaps their doctors have told them there is nothing more they can do for them or their migraine may be getting more unmanageable or their child has just been diagnosed and they do not want him or her to go through the lifetime of agony they have suffered.

The first thing to say is there is always something you can do. Migraine is very much the kind of condition that the more information you have, the more you can help yourself. Many people are suspicious of drugs and hate taking them, but if you approach medicines like this, your treatments are very likely to fail. However, there are many other things you can do that can make an impact on the management of your migraine. With correct information, self-knowledge, a medication or other treatment that works for you and a little help from colleagues and those closest to you, you could greatly reduce the severity and frequency of your attacks, if not avoid them altogether.

Finding the correct management for you can take time, but it will be time well spent. It will take time because migraine is a very complicated condition, and I hope to give you all the information you need to understand it and make informed judgements on its management and treatment. I will take you, step by step, through what is known about migraine, how to understand the clues your body gives you to enable you to cope with an attack and to achieve long-term prevention. It is not easy to understand how our bodies work and even scientists, calling on knowledge accumulated over decades, are still unsure of the exact mechanisms of a migraine.

Improvement will not happen by itself. You have to be honest with yourself, look realistically at the problem.

- What have you done so far?
- Have you really approached the search for your trigger factors properly?
- Have you kept the search up properly?
- Have you always taken your medication as instructed, at exactly the right time?
- Have you taken it for long enough?
- Did you take it at all?

A percentage of sufferers will accept a prescription for a medication, but will never take it to be filled, or else have it filled but never take it. Research that was carried out at the Princess Margaret Migraine Clinic by Catarci, et al. found, by using a specially made pill container that recorded the times it was opened, that a very large proportion of sufferers had not taken their pills in a way that would have either maximized their efficacy or made them in any way beneficial.

THE DIFFERENCE BETWEEN LIFELONG SUFFERERS AND THOSE WITH ADULT ONSET

I have often been struck by the differences in approach of those who have suffered since childhood and those who have known a 'normal' life and have then developed migraine. The lifelong sufferer definitely tends to acquiesce and accept migraine to a much greater extent. I suppose this is not surprising when you consider that they have known no other way of life, only life with migraine. Being the tremendously adaptable organisms human beings are, we adapt our lifestyle and expectations to the condition in which we find ourselves. We tend to make the best of it. Unfortunately, the lifelong sufferer can miss out on proper management because of this. Your expectations are likely to be lower. You may well believe you just have to live with it, and if you believe that, you will end up having to.

SELF-EMPOWERMENT

The responsibility for your migraine is ultimately yours. Doctors do not have all the answers or the in-depth knowledge about management that you will be able to research for yourself. This is not a negative reflection on GPs' abilities or interests, but they are general practitioners after all and their knowledge is, by definition, broad-based. Their major responsibility is correct diagnosis and your care at a primary level, to guide you along the correct road, to treat you as far as they are able and to recognize when to refer you on to a neurologist or neurologist specializing in migraine or a migraine clinic. Quite a proportion of migraine specialists are migraine sufferers themselves and so have developed their obvious interest in the condition with first-hand experience. But even a specialist, with all the knowledge of treatment, will not necessarily have all the knowledge you as a sufferer need to cope with your particular migraine.

You will notice that the chapter on management is as large as the chapter on treatment. Management is to do with how you deal with the condition yourself – what active steps you can take and the strategies you can use to ensure that your vulnerability is kept down to a minimum. Treatment involves the therapies you can use to deal with actual attacks or to minimize the frequency or severity of attacks overall. You will obviously need the treatments while you are getting to grips with the management, but the more you are able to do on the management side, the less you should need on the treatment side.

MYTHS AND REALITIES

It is always unwise to act uncritically on anecdotal advice, like the advice a neighbour who also has migraine attacks might give to you. The 'you must try so-and-so drug, it is wonderful' as he gives you a pill to try. First of all, migraine is extremely individual to each person affected. What works for one person does not necessarily work for another. If it were as easy as that, there would be no need for research, no need for different treatments or drugs and no need for this book.

Do not trust the accuracy of everything you read in newspapers or hear on the television or radio. I see first hand what happens to press releases – they are sent off and the information later appears in the Media and it has been changed. This is not to imply that the Media are malicious, aim to mislead or are negligent, but, of necessity, they have to interpret the information they receive, adapt it to their particular readership, listeners or viewers, simplify where they feel they need to, abbreviate where they must and even subtle changes can lead to the meaning being altered. Also press releases themselves can be misleading or ambiguous. Our language is complicated and some concepts are difficult to simplify well.

This does not mean that you should not pay attention to the Media. Their strength is that they can introduce a topic to you, a new piece of research, new drug on the market, new technique in management or whatever, but you should always follow it up yourself. If it comes from a news item on TV, ask them for their source and get in touch with that source. The same with a newspaper or radio programme. Alternatively, get in touch with an organization like The Migraine Trust, which follows up any new information, either to find out more or correct anything that is misleading.

What is the point of finding out more about migraine? Well, how can you make judgements about your own migraine if you have nothing to measure it against? It is important to know what you are working towards and what it is possible to achieve. It is important to put your migraine into perspective.

The history of migraine

HOW LONG HAS MIGRAINE BEEN WITH US?
One of the first images of migraine therapy that struck me was a drawing of an Egyptian with a baby alligator strapped to his head, visually describing how some Egyptians treated their migraine attacks. Although I will be giving you many ideas about management and treatment in this book, I promise you will not have to try that particular strategy!

Migraine was first described thousands of years ago. Knowing that it is a problem that people have suffered from since ancient times may give you some solace, but this also tells us that migraine is not just a reaction to the stresses of modern lifestyle and diet.

Headaches are mentioned in the Papyrus Ebers, which was written 1500BC but only discovered in a tomb in Thebes in 1862. In it is an exotic collection of prescriptions and spells to use for various medical conditions. One of our first treatments for the stubborn headache was to smear the aching head with a poultice of hide-of-hippopotamus and poppy seeds.

The Greek physician, Aretaeus of Cappadocia, who lived in Rome in the second half of the second century AD, was one of the first ever to document the condition. He wrote two treatises that have fortunately come down to us today: *On the Causes and Indications of Acute and Chronic Diseases* and *On Their Treatment* (Adams). From these we get the first really in-depth descriptions, and they indicate that migraine has hardly changed.

Galen, another Greek physician, the founder of experimental physiology, first coined the word 'hemicrania' for this condition, a word that almost certainly came from the Egyptian *gs-tp*, meaning, literally, 'half-head' (J. R. Harris). This is probably where our current term 'migraine' comes from.

Headaches are also described in Islamic literature as a disease caused by an accumulation of noxious matter.

To bear witness to the fact that having migraine does not preclude you from greatness, we know that Julius Caesar, Sigmund Freud, Joan of Arc, Lewis Carroll and Thomas Jefferson were all sufferers. In fact, it was thought that migraine sufferers were more intelligent than most people. This idea probably came about because the more educated a person was, the more likely they were to seek help for an attack and be able to access the necessary information to help manage an attack — in general a person with a higher profile. Migraine, though, touches every age, race, sex and level of intelligence.

What causes migraine?

No one yet knows exactly why migraine occurs. Research has looked at the symptoms in order to find clues as to what underlying mechanisms might explain them all. Indeed, any theory would have to explain all the typical symptoms, from what causes their various stages, why various triggers bring them on and why people of a certain age or sex are more typically prone, in fact all the varied biochemical, metabolic and neurophysiological changes that happen during an attack.

THE HYPOTHESES

We know from migraine with aura that the brain is involved, from the pain of the headache that the blood vessels are involved, from the nausea and vomiting that the gastrointestinal tract is involved. However, we do not yet have the whole picture or know in which of these systems the attack originates and which of the other systems are provoked as a consequence.

Various research findings have suggested that migraine may be a form of vascular problem, especially as the headache is usually of a throbbing type, synchronized with the pulse and it is relieved by pressure on the temporal artery. Also, vasoconstricting drugs (those that constrict the arteries) can abort attacks.

As long ago as the seventeenth century, when William Harvey had just discovered that the blood circulates around the body, Thomas Willis put forward the theory that migraine was caused by dilation of the blood vessels. Then, at the beginning of the twentieth century, Harold Wolff first studied migraine in the laboratory. He did several experiments with vasoactive drugs (ones that either distend or dilate blood vessels) and these confirmed the vascular link.

As the platelets in the blood store most of the body's serotonin, attention then turned to studying this brain chemical. It was found that some sufferers of migraine with aura had increased platelet aggregability (that is the platelets clumped together more than in people who do not get migraine), but some thought that this probably happened as a result of other factors of a migraine attack and was not the cause of it.

Advances in techniques for measuring blood flow have now shown that there is no increase of blood flow during the headache phase and that only a third of sufferers experience dilation of the temporal arteries and this, among other evidence, led away from the vascular theory being the only explanation.

This led to another theory. It suggests that migraine is a problem to do with the central nervous system originating in the brain. This is evidenced by various aspects of the visual aura and the passage and timing of its spread forwards over the visual cortex. In other tests for general pain relief, it was found that electrodes planted in the brain caused a migraine-like headache attack, which suggests that pain thresholds in migraine sufferers may be faulty in some way.

Another clue is that a quarter of sufferers experience changes in mood and appetite in the 24 hours before the headache (the prodromal phase), which suggests that the hypothalamus is involved. Evidence is now building to suggest that migraine originates in the brainstem and that it is probably due to some sort of hypersensitivity, which causes the neurological and vascular symptoms.

However, it was still not understood what caused the blood vessels to react. Research was done into the neurotransmitters (chemical messengers) of the body, which were known to affect the blood vessels. The previously mentioned serotonin, also known as 5-hydroxytryptamine or 5-HT, was found to be the most interesting of these as 5-HT levels were shown to briefly rise during the aura stage but then fall dramatically during the headache stage. Attacks could also be triggered by taking substances that reduce 5-HT levels or aborted by giving 5-HT intravenously.

This has led to a further theory; that migraine is a molecular dysfunction. 5-HT, which happens to be naturally present in the brain, is implicated in blood vessels, in the gastrointestinal tract and in blood platelets. This has led pharmaceutical companies to develop a new generation of 5-HT agonist drugs and these have been found to be very effective in aborting migraine attacks.

Other molecules that are thought to be involved in migraine are also being researched. There are many questions that have been answered, but many questions that still need to be asked.

THE GENETIC BASIS OF MIGRAINE

Because of modern technical advances, the study of the genetic basis of migraine has become possible. What most sufferers will be familiar with is a tendency for migraine to run in families. How many of you have parents, siblings or children who also suffer? However, there was no direct genetic evidence to underpin the theory that there is a genetic mode of transmission.

Study at the molecular level started in earnest in 1993 with a French study of two large families (Joutel, et al.), published in Nature, linking Familial Hemiplegic Migraine, a rarer form of migraine, to chromosome 19. Since then, cluster headache has also been shown to have a genetic basis.

From this and other work, it looks as though, in the not too distant future, the actual gene sequence responsible for migraine will be identified. With this knowledge will come the possibility of testing for migraine, which will have wide-reaching consequences for the treatment of the condition. It will revolutionize the way many in the medical profession think about migraine as there will be a test to identify it – like diabetes or high blood pressure – as a tangible condition. It will have to be taken seriously.

It will also mean that it will be possible to identify the exact mechanism of the migraine in any one individual and, hence, identify what would be the best treatment in that particular case, especially which drug will be effective. At the moment, it is a hit-and-miss affair, sufferers trying one drug after another in their sometimes weary and demoralizing search for one that works for them.

Finally, it opens up the possibility that, at some point in the future, we may be able to 'cure' migraine by means of genetic engineering, when this branch of medicine has developed sufficiently.

Frequency

The average number of days people suffer from migraine is about one a month for about 62 per cent of all sufferers. This means that, happily, the majority of sufferers do not have to tolerate the condition too often. However, this still leaves a large proportion of sufferers – well over a quarter – who suffer them more often. The worst sufferers, many of whom make up a large part of The Migraine Trust's membership, can suffer them two or three times a week.

PREVALENCE AND DISTRIBUTION

How common is migraine? Of the 100 or so types of headaches, migraine and tension headaches are the most prevalent. Statistics have varied greatly, indicating that between 5 and 35 per cent of the population of the world suffer from them. However, many population studies carried out in the past have been based on biased sampling, that is, not studying migraine sufferers from among the general population, but from groups such as doctor's referrals, clinics and so on and, by definition, these groups are likely to include a high proportion of severe and chronic cases. Specific criteria for diagnosing migraine were introduced and generally adopted in 1988 so we now know that in the more recent studies the same criteria are being used in each case for diagnosing migraine and certainly the figures from these studies are tending to agree more closely than before these criteria were being used. Figures also vary according to whether you look at prevalence over a year or two or over a lifetime, which can also give quite varied results. Taking this into account, the general prevalence over any one year is now recognized to be about 10 per cent, that is, one in ten people suffer (6 per cent of men and 15 per cent of women). The figures for lifetime prevalence are as high as 16 per cent (one in twelve men and one in four women – a quarter of all women!) As you can see, this means that the incidence of women sufferers is three times greater than for men. It affects *a quarter of all women* and yet the public health significance of this is still unrecognized.

Migraine seems to be suffered by all communities and cultures. Research studies have been carried out on specific communities – high school students, Turkish women, Australian twins, Zulu tribespeople, Swedish primary school children. Lipton, et al. (1994) cites 58 population-based migraine prevalence studies. The results show that there seems to be no particular pattern to the type, age, gender, class or ethnic origin of a person who is prone to migraine.

THE SIGNIFICANCE OF MIGRAINE

Given the size of the problem, why is migraine not regarded as more of a serious health issue? The major reasons for this may be that attacks are benign – you do not die from them – and they are episodic – they come and go. This means that, although you may be severely disabled by migraine during an actual attack, you are perfectly normal between attacks. Also, there is no test for migraine yet. The only tests which may be done are those carried out in order to preclude other conditions so, in a way, it is not easy to quantify migraine. The public health implications are therefore considered minor and less than 0.1 per cent of the national health budget is spent on them.

Despite this lack of recognition, it has been projected that the average number of days sufferers are absent from work a year due to migraine is about six for men and about seven for women (Cull, *et al.*, 1992). Multiply that by the number of sufferers – 6 million in the UK, 120 million worldwide – and you will begin to appreciate just what an impact the condition must have on productivity in industry. Research into migraine and how to alleviate its effect would therefore seem an ideal area for industry to support.

2

THE ATTACK

What is migraine?

If you would prefer a more scientific description of migraine than a recurring biological timebomb, it can be described clinically as an episodic primary headache disorder – 'primary' because there is no other underlying disease causing the condition and 'episodic' because they come and go and there is complete freedom from the problem between attacks.

TYPICAL CHARACTERISTICS OF MIGRAINE
Typical characteristics of the headache aspect are that it is commonly one-sided (unilateral), although a third of headaches affect both sides, and they are often pulsating or throbbing in quality, of moderate to severe intensity (although it tends to be milder in children) and it can be aggravated by physical exertion.

There is usually a history of a close family (blood) relative suffering too (a familial tendency).

A migraine attack can last between 4 and 72 hours (although in children it tends to be shorter). Nearly always it features a headache and some sort of stomach disorder or, more correctly, disorder of the gastrointestinal tract. Nausea is the most typical symptom of this, although occasionally vomiting, anorexia, diarrhoea or constipation are experienced. There is also a hypersensitivity to light (photophobia) and sound (phonophobia). There can also be a variety of neurological symptoms.

These are the basic symptoms, behind which lie a myriad of others that go to make migraine such a complicated but fascinating illness, as well as one which is so difficult to define.

From my repetition of the phrases 'usually is', 'can be' and 'often is', you will have realized that migraine is not a condition that can be precisely described. The above symptoms are typical features of an attack, each one to be ticked off a mental 'checklist' and, when sufficient symptoms are present, contributing towards a positive diagnosis.

For example, when I say the headache is 'often pulsating', I am saying that a typical quality of a migraine headache, as opposed to some other type of headache, is that it is a pulsating one. In fact, though, a large proportion of migraine headaches are not pulsating. You may be just as likely to have an aching headache or you may have first one sort then another during the same attack or else one sort during one attack, and another sort during another. However, this said, if it is pulsating, it counts towards a positive diagnosis of migraine.

Problems with diagnosis

There can be trouble diagnosing migraine, especially migraine without aura. This can not only make life difficult for doctors, but also for research purposes, leading to research findings that have been difficult to replicate or wildly differing in results, as one group defines certain symptoms as migranous and another group does not.

THE INTERNATIONAL HEADACHE SOCIETY CRITERIA

Fortunately, in 1988, an *ad hoc* committee of The International Headache Society drew up a set of classification and diagnostic criteria that have become the basis for diagnoses throughout the world. By means of this checklist, a recognizable standard definition of a migraine has been achieved. I have included the entry for migraine on page 127, which will give you some idea as to why the doctor asks you all those odd questions.

The incidence figures of 1 in 4 women and 1 in 12 men suffering from migraine are now based on this recognized standard, in that diagnoses are made according to it, are, in fact, highly conservative (that is they are an absolute minimum) because it is used for research purposes. The *actual* incidence of migraine is probably two to three times higher than this. When sufferers say their migraine make them feel so isolated and alone, perhaps it will help to remember this fact, and know that they are far from being alone.

ARE ALL YOUR HEADACHES MIGRAINE?

Many migraine sufferers also experience other headaches (usually tension-type headaches) between their migraine attacks – sometimes referred to as 'mixed headaches'. It is important to identify these as being different as the management and treatment of each type can be different. In fact, some sufferers may develop daily headaches if they take medications incorrectly. So, get your doctor to diagnose them. Also, read about how to identify the different headaches and how to control each of them because, as I have mentioned, they each may need different management.

CONFIRMING THE DIAGNOSIS

However typical you think your symptoms are, you must always have your diagnosis confirmed by a doctor. This is because some symptoms can also be indicative of other disorders. Of all doctor's consultations, 60 per cent will include headache as a symptom.

Only doctors have sufficient knowledge of what factors are significant. They are trained to spot symptoms of other conditions that may be coexisting with your migraine and, if they do, these other conditions must be treated as well. A doctor's input can also be very helpful – in some cases crucial – to successful management of migraine. In most cases, the diagnosis will be straightforward.

Patients sometimes feel that they should be sent for tests and that their doctors are not bothering enough if they do not do so, but there is actually no test you can do at the moment that will indicate whether or not you have migraine (although, as mentioned earlier, this looks to be on the horizon). Diagnoses can be adequately made from a careful history taken by a doctor in the majority of cases. It is only if the doctor is unsure of the diagnosis that you may be sent for tests. These can include brain scans, such as a CT (computer tomography) or MRI scan (magnetic resonance imaging), skull X-ray, EEG (electroencephalogram) or lumbar puncture, depending on what your symptoms suggest. However, the tests are not primarily to confirm migraine, but to exclude other illnesses.

A portrait of migraine

Mary had been feeling very tired and uneasy the whole of the previous day. That morning she had struggled to dress her two young children and take them out shopping. As she was waiting to cross the road outside the supermarket, the shop in front of her suddenly disappeared.

She looked down at her children, but couldn't see them. The aura of a migraine attack was starting. She felt panic. Her daughter was saying something to her but she felt confused. She turned to a woman beside her in desperation to ask her for help, but the words came out in a jumble, and the woman gave her an odd look and hurried away. She started shaking uncontrollably and her eyes began to stream. All she could think of was that she must keep tight hold of her children. She was holding her son's hand so tightly he had started to cry.

Mary managed to struggle home. By the time she got there, some of her missing vision had returned, but a throbbing pain was building up on the right side of her head, and a strong feeling of nausea gripped her stomach. She fumbled as she tried to get the key in the lock, got inside with the children and collapsed on the settee.

Half an hour later and the headache was excruciating. The children, as they had been left to their own devices, were running about noisily. Every sound felt like a screech in her head, but she couldn't move because it made the pain and nausea worse. Fortunately her neighbour came round and, seeing the situation she had come to know so well, offered to look after the children. Mary started to vomit and continued on and off for hours until finally, exhausted, she fell into a deep sleep. When she awoke, she was relieved to find that the headache had gone, but it took her another full day to recover properly.

Even on a normal day, whenever she went out with the children she felt occasional waves of fear in case she had a migraine attack while she was out and somehow was not able to look after them. It was a fear she never lost until they were old enough to look after themselves. That part was even worse than the pain she felt during the attacks.

Fortunately, not all migraine sufferers' attacks are as bad as this, but it should underline the fact that migraine is far removed from being just a headache. Over the years I have heard so many different recollections of the pain, the fear of an attack and the devastation of normal life.

The stages of an attack

NOT JUST A HEADACHE

So many people think exclusively of the headache when thinking of migraine – that is, unless you are a sufferer. Then you are only too aware of the many and often disconcerting, sometimes alarming biological changes that take place during an attack. These seem to fall into distinct stages, although even these can overlap. Blau (1982) has suggested dividing what happens during an attack into five stages:

- prodromal – also called premonitory, or warning, signs
- aura
- headache
- resolution
- postdromal or recovery – the aftermath or 'hangover' period.

This does help to give a strong mental image of migraine as being an attack moving through time – through the first subtle changes, developing, reaching a climax and subsiding until it reaches its conclusion, moving *from* normality *back* to normality.

All five stages need not be evident in a migraine attack. One individual might only have the prodromal and headache stages. Another may have no prodromal or aura stages, just the headache, resolution and aftermath. Some just have the aura, with none of the other stages (more common in older sufferers). These patterns may vary from individual to individual and also from attack to attack. Nonetheless, the headache nearly always seems to be the focus of most attacks, even if the headache is not always the aspect that is the most disturbing or the most disabling.

Premonitory, or warning, signs

At the beginning of the migraine attack, certain physical and mental changes can occur. Their onset may be an hour or two before the headache or up to a day or two before – they vary enormously from person to person and need not always be the same symptoms from one attack to another. Mostly they are vague – sometimes so vague that sufferers themselves are not aware of them, only their friends or family notice them – yet studies done have identified them in between 40 and 80 per cent of sufferers.

Sometimes they are quite pronounced or there is just a general feeling of being not quite right, but it is difficult to specify exactly why. Here is a list of some that have been noted, just to give you an idea of the breadth of symptoms:

* changes in mood or behaviour
* dizziness
* irritability
* loss of concentration
* depression
* fear
* unusual pallor
* elation
* trembling
* exaggerated feeling of wellbeing
* weakness, especially of the muscles
* excitability
* tingling sensations
* fatigue or lethargy
* numbness
* yawning
* neck stiffness or pain
* hyperactivity and unusual amounts of energy

- increased bowel or bladder activity
- slurred speech
- increase in weight
- swollen fingers, breasts or waist
- slow thinking
- hunger or craving for a particular food, often sweet things
- blotchy skin or rash
- sensitivity to light (photophonia)
- nausea
- sensitivity to sound (phonophobia)
- loss of appetite
- feeling cold
- vomiting
- difficulty in speaking
- thirst
- double vision, partial loss of vision or visual disturbances
- memory loss
- difficulty in focusing
- obsessional behaviour.

You can see that many of these symptoms are excitatory or inhibitory symptoms, representing a speeding up or slowing down of different senses or processes. They do not start suddenly, but build up over time. You may experience one, two or more. Often, if you experience a premonitory symptom, such as craving for food, you may have the reverse, a loss of appetite, towards the end of the attack, like the reverse swing of a pendulum.

The premonitory symptoms are sometimes mistaken for triggers. You may be overtired, and this triggers a migraine attack. Or feeling tired is the first sign of a migraine attack; the first stage as it were. Treatments started at this stage are more likely to be effective.

The aura

The *Oxford English Dictionary* (1994) describes 'aura' as 'distinctive atmosphere – subtle emanation'. Dorland's medical dictionary explains it as 'a peculiar sensation forerunning the appearance of more definite symptoms'. This is rather an inadequate description of this particular phase, which has caused such interest among researchers because of its unusual and fascinating symptoms. If this stage is present in an attack, by definition you will be experiencing *migraine with aura*.

The aura is a complex of neurological symptoms thought to be caused by regional blood flow changes in the brain, originating in the brainstem. This has been termed cortical spreading depression – 'depression' here meaning a constriction of blood flow that gradually spreads forwards across the cerebral cortex. It is thought that as the depression moves forwards, so different areas of the cortex are affected, which can give rise to the several different types of aura. All auras are themselves developing phenomena, involving movement in time and space.

The descriptions available of the aura symptoms are few and imprecise, given by patients in clinics, usually describing them retrospectively, or drawn from patient records or sufferers responses to questionnaires. Some of the most rigorous descriptions have been given by sufferers who are doctors or scientists themselves, describing the various effects as they were happening. It has been suggested, however, that even they may have been a little biased, paying greater attention to the more interesting symptoms.

The aura need not be visual, although this is the most well known and certainly the most common form. There are also sensory, speech (dysphasic) and motor auras or combinations of these – motor auras being the rarest. If only one aura is apparent, then it will almost certainly be the visual one. When more than one is evident, then it is usually the visual plus sensory, speech and/or motor occurring one after the other, never together. It has been suggested that this is due to the movement of the wave of constriction of blood flow as it moves from one area of the brain to the next. The phenomena are very varied, involving changes in physical and emotional states and distortions of reality. There can be overall changes in your sensory threshold when sensory experiences are heightened and then reduced below normal.

The aura mainly occurs between 5 to 30 minutes before the headache. The average duration is about 20 minutes. Occasionally it can accompany the headache, while in rarer cases it can outlast it for hours or days. If you do experience aura, you will not necessarily experience it during every attack. Strangely, migraine attacks with aura tend to be more intense, but much shorter.

Visual aura

The visual disturbances can include hallucinations of great variety; flashing lights, starbursts, zigzag patterns, scotoma (holes in the visual field or blind spots), blurring or even loss of vision, shining lines, constellation or fortification patterns, in fact myriad symptoms, with no two experiences being exactly alike. It has been suggested that visual aura are caused by disturbances of the occipital cortex, although, interestingly, visual hallucinations like these have not been replicated by stimulating the brain artificially.

Here is one person's description of their experience of an aura, including a scotoma and typical fortification spectra.

I was watching a cricket match on the television and began to realize that I was confused about what was happening on the pitch. I just couldn't understand what was going on, until I realized the reason was

*because I could not see the left-hand side of the screen until I angled
my head to the left and looked at the screen from the right-hand side.
I suddenly realized there was no visual information coming back from
that area. As I stared directly ahead, there was a blank patch, centre
left, slightly bottom left of my vision. The only way to describe it was
like a large ink blot, but not black or dark, but a greeny grey or neu-
tral area. It was not a 'black out' but a 'grey out'.*

*Very quickly after this I became aware of an irregular saw-tooth
crescent-shaped neon light, as if it was a faulty tube, which flickered
on and off in the left-hand bottom side of my vision, and this went on
flickering for about ten minutes. The saw-tooth shape was not all
bright — it had dark parts between. After this the crescent got fainter
and it was replaced by a violent headache focused above the eyes. If
this is a migraine, I suspect I have had it many times before, as I have
had the same kind of headache, when you feel really frightened to
move your head because of the intensity of the pain, but I have only
experienced the visual aura twice in my life, no nausea at all, and the
first time, which was about 18 months ago, I experienced only the
visual symptoms, but they were not followed by a headache.*

Other sensory aura

The second most common aura gives rise to limb symptoms,
such as tingling or a sensation of pins and needles. These will
usually start in the hand, most commonly the tip of a finger or
thumb, and spread up the arm to the face, mouth and/or
tongue. Occasionally the leg and foot can be similarly affected.
The tingling sensation is usually superseded by numbness and
eventually even a loss of sense of position of the affected limb.

There may be stranger sensory hallucinations, such as feeling that your arms are growing longer, your neck is stretching,
distortions of your physical sense of self. You may also experience distortions of reality, feelings of strangeness, abstraction
or fear, distortions of memory.

Speech can also be affected, when the sufferer experiences aphasia (an inability to pronounce words or name objects) or dysarthria (an impairment of the ability to speak). You can know exactly what you want to say, but cannot find the words or the right order in which to say them. One sufferer attempted to leave a written message for a visitor who was coming round to her house while she was out, but found she could not. Although she tried several times, she knew the note was not making sense, but she did not know why. After the migraine attacks had finished, she reread the note and found that the right words were there, but in all the wrong order, some even repeated, but she had spelt the words correctly, even the more complicated ones.

More rarely, sufferers experience a sense of weakness on one side, such as temporary partial paralysis, vertigo or loss of consciousness. Oliver Sacks gives an in-depth exploration of the complexities of aura in his book on migraine.

The headache

The headache stage involves not only a headache, but other accompanying symptoms. There is invariably a disturbance of the gastrointestinal tract, which most commonly causes either nausea and, less frequently, vomiting.

Site and intensity

The headache of a migraine can be of a moderate to severe intensity, sometimes totally incapacitating, and lying down in a darkened room seems to be the only way of coping with it. It usually starts as a general awareness of the head and slowly progresses from mild, building up to medium and then severe pain, although the speed with which this happens does vary from person to person. The headache can be throbbing (if it is, it fulfills one of the criteria for a positive diagnosis of a migraine), but it could just as well be a pressing or tightening pain. The pain is aggravated by movement, especially bending down, which often brings on the throbbing pain. This is often relieved by pressure on the temporal artery, which is at the side of the temple.

Migraine is typically unilateral (one-sided), especially at its onset. However, they can also be bilateral, especially over the forehead. It is rarer to experience a headache at the back of the head; this is more likely to be tension headache, which can occur between migraine attacks in many sufferers.

The teeth, shoulder, neck and eye of one side can be affected, often mimicking sinusitis. Some people always experience headaches on the same side, while for others the site changes from one side to the other in different attacks or during the same attack or is sometimes one-sided and sometimes not.

Duration

The International Headache Society criteria gives a headache duration time of from 4 to 72 hours, although in children it has been suggested that this should be revised to 2 hours as a minimum, as headaches in children seem to be shorter and less intense than in adults.

The resolution

The headache and accompanying symptoms may just fade away in time or resolve themselves as a result of taking medication or some other active treatment. It may also be resolved violently, by vomiting or copious weeping or aborted by sleep, the latter being one of the most common and effective 'treatments'. Even a brief sleep can be effective. Eating can also effectively abort an attack if it was caused by your body's reaction to lack of food.

The recovery

The fact that this stage is a 'recovery' stage implies, of course, that all is not over, which is indeed the case. There is often an aftermath or 'hangover' after the headache has gone. The length of the recovery stage is usually between an hour or two and up to one day, but it can drag on for three or four days. This stage is often overlooked or ignored by both clinicians and literature; maybe there have been enough of the other various and fascinating symptoms going before to keep them fully absorbed. Also, the fact that the worst of the attack has finished perhaps overshadows the significance of this lingering stage, but it is very significant to the person who experiences it, especially if they are a frequent sufferer.

As mentioned at the beginning of the chapter, many of the premonitory symptoms can be mirrored at this stage of the attack. For example, you may be constipated, lethargic or lack concentration at the beginning of an attack and have diarrhoea, an enormous amount of energy or be extremely alert at the end of an attack. As you may not have been able to face much food before, because of the nausea and vomiting, you may feel ravenous now and lightheaded from a lack of food; try having light meals if your stomach is still not back to normal. There may have been a period of fluid retention at the beginning of the attack; there could now be heavy urination, releasing the build-up of fluid. If there was constipation before, there could now be a period of diarrhoea and stomach ache.

Sometimes there are no obvious links with the start of the attack. Many people experience lethargy and aching all over the body with muscle weakness. It can sometimes be a positive experience, a time of high achievement and inventiveness, if you are lucky.

Between attacks

It has long been thought that a migraine suffer has a natural immunity to migraine just after an attack. This would make sense if we accept that, by definition, there is complete freedom from attacks between one attack and the next. However, research done by Dr de Belleroche in London, funded by The Migraine Trust, found that the pathways of transmission of messages between one cell and another were impaired in migraine sufferers, not only during migraine attacks, but between attacks, which points to a predisposition to attacks in sufferers.

Changing patterns

Not only does migraine vary from individual to individual and from attack to attack in the same individual, patterns can also change with age and circumstance.

AGE OF ONSET

Migraine has been reported in those as young as 1 year old, but the average age of onset is 19 and 90 per cent of sufferers have experienced their first attack before the age of 40. Then, the older you get, the more likely it is that you will never have an attack. If you develop migraine in childhood, you have a 50:50 chance of growing out of it by the time you become an adult.

CHILDHOOD

Patterns of attack in children are usually different to adults. The major symptom in childhood tends to be stomach-related, that is, stomach ache or pain and nausea, with the headache tending to be less severe. If a child has severe headache, you should seek medical advice. Attacks also tend to be shorter. A two-hour attack is not unusual, whereas the adult attack is rarely shorter than four. Children seem to be particularly sensitive to missing a meal or not getting enough sleep. Sleep itself is often the best treatment for the young migraine sufferer, even a brief sleep often aborts an attack. As the nature and treatment of migraine can be different, I have given it a whole section to itself later on in the book.

PUBERTY

As younger sufferers reach puberty, although half grow out of their migraine and go on to be migraine-free throughout their adult lives, the other half continue to suffer. However, the pattern of attack usually changes at this time and the headache symptom can now become the most dominant.

Puberty can also trigger migraine in those who have not experienced it before, especially girls. The ratio of female to male in childhood is roughly equal, but after puberty, the ratio goes up to 3 girls to every 1 boy. This has been interpreted as indicating that the role of female hormones in migraine is significant. Indeed, between 50 and 70 per cent of women sufferers are convinced that their migraine are closely linked to their menstrual cycles. Also, the fact that women's patterns of attack often change in line with their reproductive lives – that is, they typically start during puberty, improve during pregnancy and can worsen at menopause – seems to uphold this. However, Lipton and Stewart's study of migraine in the US shows there to be only a small reduction in the sex ratio in those over 70. Also women who typically suffer menstrual migraine (that is, their migraine attacks occur only at the beginning of menstruation, plus or minus two or three days), can continue to follow the same pattern even after their periods have ceased, which implies that the link is not that straightforward.

ADULTHOOD

In adulthood, as mentioned, the headache tends to become the major symptom of an attack. Apart from those women who suffer true menstrual migraine — only having attacks at the time of their menstruation — women can have attacks triggered at the start of menstruation and at mid-cycle as well, probably corresponding to ovulation. Here a hormonal link looks evident.

Women also find that they may be immune to particular triggers at certain times of their menstrual cycle and not others. For example, if cheese is a trigger, they may be able to eat it just after their menstruation without effect, but not just before, when they are prone to attack.

PREGNANCY

Pregnancy brings an improvement in the pattern of attacks or complete relief for nearly three quarters of women sufferers, especially for those whose attacks are closely linked to their hormonal cycles. However, for a small percentage of unlucky women, it is aggravated by pregnancy, especially in the first three months. If you are so affected, see page 118 for how to deal with the problems of management and treatment in pregnancy and while breastfeeding.

For about 10 per cent of women, their attack patterns remain the same as they were before they became pregnant. Headaches can also occur or worsen just after the baby has been born, but the migraine quickly reverts to its pre-pregnancy patterns. Also, occasionally, pregnancy can bring about the onset of migraine. Occasionally, too, a sufferer who previously experienced migraine without aura has migraine with aura for the first time while pregnant.

THE MENOPAUSE

It is well established that migraine resolves itself with age, yet some women who still have migraine when they are older can find that their migraine actually worsens at this time, especially where their hormones are a triggering factor.

Occasionally a woman who has previously suffered from menstrual migraine may continue to have migraine at the same time each month even though their periods have ceased. It has also been suggested that the loss of sleep as a result of the various menopausal symptoms, such as night sweats or inability to sleep, can itself trigger more headaches than usual. Once the menopause has finished the migraine should improve.

HRT AND THE PILL

Occasionally starting to take oral contraceptives can correspond with a woman's first experience of migraine, and there is supporting evidence to suggest that these events are linked. In the majority of cases, oral contraceptives have no effect on migraine patterns. For some, attacks improve. If one type of oral contraceptive does cause you problems, though, there are other types that can be tried which will be tolerated.

In a very small percentage of cases, migraine without aura change into migraine with aura and if this happens, it is very important to discuss this with your doctor *immediately* as this change could indicate serious side-effects. Also see your doctor if you develop daily headaches or experience headaches that come on suddenly, rather than the usual build-up of pain. Any change in pattern should be reported to your doctor in any case.

WHAT TO DO WHEN YOUR PATTERNS CHANGE

Although you should not be alarmed by a change in pattern, as it is quite common, you must always consult your doctor to eliminate other underlying causes, especially if your attacks get worse or unusual symptoms occur. This is a sensible precaution.

3

THE HEADACHES

There are, in all, about a hundred or so types of headache —
hunger headaches, those caused by blood pressure, trauma
headaches and so on. Migraine and cluster headache are vascular headaches belonging to one of the major groups. Tension-
type and muscle contraction headaches make up another major
group. The headaches I mention in this chapter are those that
are likely to be of most interest to a migraine sufferer. The last
two groups, the inflammatory headaches — some benign like
sinusitis and others more serious such as meningitis and trac-
tion headaches such as brain tumours — are extremely rare. All
headaches, though, should be diagnosed by a medical expert.
It is always wise to check with your doctor if the pattern of
your headaches changes, but the chances of your headaches
being of a more serious nature are remote and the same as that
of any non-migraine sufferer.

The different types of migraine

Having a precise name for the type of migraine suffered seems
to be very important to a sufferer, even if the management or
treatment for the particular type is no different to that for any

other. Perhaps giving it a name helps acknowledge its existence, makes it more tangible. You can read about it and compare your symptoms with those given in books. There may be more to it than this, though, as the fact that certain drugs only work for certain people does indicate that different mechanisms are at work.

Sometimes a doctor will give your migraine symptoms a particular name. In fact, you can 'translate' all the medical terms for the different types mentioned later. For example, with hemiplegic migraine, the 'hemi' means 'half' and 'plegia' means 'paralysis' and, in this case, it is a form of migraine attack where one of the symptoms experienced is temporary partial paralysis on one side of the body.

Even if you are given a name for your type of migraine, bear in mind that the cause of migraine has not yet been found and there is research going on now that is even questioning whether or not migraine without aura and migraine with aura are two different entities. We therefore do not really know whether or not the different symptoms are caused by different mechanisms. It may be more helpful overall to think of migraine as a continuum – one single entity that affects different people in different ways, just as a single virus causes different symptoms in different people.

Clinicians need to use classifications to help with diagnosis and research. In Figure 2 (see page 160) you will see the International Headache Society's criteria for migraine.

You can see from this that the International Headache Society classifies migraine into seven main divisions. If you have been told you suffer from *basilar migraine*, you can see from the box that you actually suffer from a subtype of *migraine with aura* and, in this case, the symptoms that typify basilar migraine, like difficulty in speaking and feeling dizzy, are part of the aura. Thus a doctor uses the name to diagnose, but in a way it is only a description of particular symptoms typical to your experience of migraine.

Here are descriptions of the major ones to help you understand the terms and the symptoms the names used represent.

MIGRAINE WITHOUT AURA

This is the most widespread form of migraine. About 70 per cent of migraine sufferers have this type. It was formerly called *common migraine* or *hemicrania simplex*. The International Headache Society describes it as an idiopathic (occurring without a known cause), recurring headache disorder manifesting in attacks lasting 4 to 72 hours. Typical characteristics are unilateral (one-sided) location, pulsating quality, moderate to severe intensity, aggravated by routine activity and associated with nausea, photo- and phonophobia (sensitivity to light and sound). A full description is given under The stages of an attack, page 19, but without the aura stage.

MIGRAINE WITH AURA

This was previously called *classic* or *classical migraine, ophthalmic* (not ophthalmoplegic, which is given below), *hemiplegic* or *aphasic migraine, hemiparesthetic migraine, complicated migraine* or *migraine accompagnée*.

This type can have all the characteristics of migraine without aura, with the addition of the aura stage. Full details of a typical attack are given under The stages of an attack, page 19.

This form is experienced by about 30 per cent of migraine sufferers. If you suffer from migraine with aura, you may sometimes experience migraine without aura, but rarely the other way round. One form has been known to transform into the other (*transformed migraine*), even after years of suffering exclusively from one form.

Migraine with typical aura, is self-explanatory. The aura of a migraine may very occasionally last longer than an hour and this might then be classified as *migraine with prolonged aura*. It can go on for days. Sufferers rarely experience this, but, if they do, its occurrence is occasionally within other more typical attacks. Consult your doctor if you experience this for the first time.

MIGRAINE AURA WITHOUT HEADACHE

I often come across sufferers who experience the visual disturbances of migraine without the headache. This seems to happen particularly with older sufferers, who will usually cite a previous lifetime history of migraine with aura. However, even though the visual disturbance is thoroughly familiar to them, it seems to be very disturbing when the familiar headache is not there with it. In fact, it seems to be more troublesome than the headache as it prevents them carrying on a normal life. It may also occur more often than their normal migraine attacks did before.

HEMIPLEGIC MIGRAINE

Hemiplegic migraine is a form of migraine that involves hemiparesis, which means partial temporary paralysis affecting one side of the body – mostly an arm and/or leg, less commonly the head or face. The attack usually involves headache, which can go on for much longer than is usual in migraine (it may be from five to ten days).

Sickness is infrequent. It may be two or three days into the headache before a feeling of weakness starts, which gradually becomes more profound, reaches a peak and gradually recovers over the period of a week or two. There can also be confusion and drowsiness at the height of an attack.

Hemiplegic migraine is further subdivided into *familial hemiplegic migraine*, where one of your closest (first degree) blood relatives also suffers, and *non-familial hemiplegic migraine* where this is not the case.

Hemiplegic migraine is rare, although this is no consolation to those who suffer from it. Even for those who experience it, the number of migraine attacks when hemiplegia is present is likely to be small, which may be some consolation.

BASILAR MIGRAINE

Also known as *basilar artery migraine, Bickerstaff's migraine* and *syncopal migraine*, this is basically migraine with aura but with additional aura symptoms. They last about the same length of time as the conventional aura and are thought to originate (as the name implies) in the basilar artery (a blood vessel at the back of the neck at the base of the brain).

It is thought that this form of migraine is caused by temporary disturbances due to a diminished supply of blood to the brain, which is supplied by the basilar artery.

The additional symptoms can start with disturbances of the vision, which are usually scintillating scotoma or greyouts or double vision followed by difficulty in speaking, but the sufferer usually still makes sense. There may be impairment of hearing or tinnitus, too, which can affect both ears and cause an unsteadiness when walking. The patient can also experience a tingling sensation in their hands and feet, around the mouth and sometimes extending to the tongue. There is occasionally an alteration or loss of consciousness (syncope). Many of these symptoms are the same as those that can also occur as a result of anxiety or hyperventilation. The headache is of shorter duration than the norm but does not usually extend over a day.

It affects all ages, both sexes and is often seen in children. There is nearly always a history of migraine in the family of basilar migraine sufferers, although these others have not usually had migraine of the basilar type.

ABDOMINAL MIGRAINE

Some clinicians dislike the term *abdominal migraine*. You will notice that the International Headache Society classification does not mention it.

This is a form of migraine where the major symptom is not a headache, but gastrointestinal disturbance, such as a stomach ache. Children usually suffer from this type, although some adults do too, but much less commonly.

There is a more complete explanation of migraine in childhood and its treatment on page 52.

OPHTHALMOPLEGIC MIGRAINE

This, as mentioned, should not be mistaken for *ophthalmic* migraine, which means migraine in which visual symptoms constitute a significant component of the attack.

Ophthalmoplegic migraine affects the oculomotor nerve, which regulates eye movements. It is most common in childhood and then affects mostly boys in the ratio 6:1.

The oculomotor nerve supplies muscles in and around the eye, including those responsible for altering the size of the pupil and those that turn the eye in different directions. The attack starts with pain in or around one eye and, as the pain increases, it spreads. This lasts for about two to ten days. Around the peak of the pain, the affected eyelid droops (ptosis) and can be accompanied by double vision (diplopia). Complete recovery can take one or two weeks.

MENSTRUAL MIGRAINE

If the vast majority of your migraine attacks occur at the start of menstruation, plus or minus two or three days, it may be that you have what is termed 'true' *menstrual migraine* although this definition is not yet recognized in the International Headache Society's criteria.

Menstrual migraine is thought to be caused by the sudden rapid drop in oestrogen levels just before the onset of menstruation. An adhesive oestradiol skin patch has been developed that you place on the thigh about three days before menstruation is due to start. It helps to prevent this drop of oestrogen being too sudden, hopefully preventing a migraine attack being triggered. It is an effective method of treatment and has the added benefit of leaving the menstrual cycle unchanged. For the treatment to be successful, however, you must have regular periods as you have to know when your period is due to be able to apply the patch at the correct time.

OTHER MIGRAINE CLASSIFICATIONS

There are other rarer forms of migraine that do not fit the International Headache Society's criteria. They can be attacks where symptoms are not fully reversible in the timescale suggested. For example, *complicated migraine* (also known as *migraine accompagnée*) is a form of migraine in which neurological deficits are present and sometimes outlast the headache. *Migraine equivalent* is where there is no headache symptom present in an attack. *Migraine infarction* is migraine where the aura symptoms outlast the attack. Indeed, it is not unknown for this to go on for a week, sometimes longer. *Status migrainous* is another form of migraine where there seems to be no period of normality between attacks. This may be due to the medications being used. The term is sometimes mistakenly used when there are tension or chronic daily headaches coexisting with migraine.

These rarer forms of migraine are best treated by specialists as they will have greater knowledge of treating them than GPs.

Other types of headache

Other headaches can coexist with migraine. It is important to identify these as they often respond to different treatments. In some instances, migraine cannot be treated until the other headache has been successfully treated.

TENSION-TYPE HEADACHE

Tension-type headache is the most common form there is. The headache is typically tight or heavy, affecting the whole of the head and often called hatband headache as the pain has been likened to a tight band being tied around the head.

The ache is constant and can last all day, every day. It varies in intensity from a slight awareness of tightness, to quite moderate pain. Movement does not effect it, but tiredness may do and, consequently, rest will often improve it. There is no nausea involved and it is not exacerbated by movement.

These headaches are often due to anxiety or depression that, in a migraine sufferer, could not unreasonably be linked with the stress and worry of living with the condition of migraine. If this is the cause, treatment includes making lifestyle changes and changes in routine to reduce stress and workload. If treatment is effective, this can not only bring about reduction in the incidence of the tension-type head-aches, but, consequently, a reduction in the frequency and severity of the migraine attacks. Conversely, taking positive steps in migraine management can also reduce tension-type headaches, as the underlying cause of the stress reduces.

Treatment of the attack is usually by analgesics. For more frequent or severe attacks, the doctor can prescribe a mild sedative for short-term use where the cause is a one-off stressor, such as a bereavement. However, the underlying cause should always be addressed.

There is some evidence that the distinction between migraine and tension-type headache may not always be valid. Research has shown that the same biochemical changes occur during both types of headache, but opinion about this is divided.

MUSCLE CONTRACTION HEADACHE

Headaches can occur as a reaction to over-stressing particular parts of the body, such as by adopting poor posture or suffering eye strain. These headaches will usually resolve themselves when the cause is removed. For example, if you stop slouching at your desk or rest your eyes periodically if you are spending prolonged sessions at the computer or VDU. More instant relief can be achieved by massage or applying a hot water bottle to the affected muscles.

DAILY HEADACHE

A lesser known headache syndrome, now found to be increasingly common, is *chronic daily headache* (CDH). This has been called 'the hidden epidemic' by Professor Edmeads, a leading migraine specialist. The Princess Margaret Migraine Clinic in London has reported that one in ten of patients attending for what was thought to be worsening migraine attacks were actually suffering from CDH.

Chronic daily headache, as its name implies, is a daily or near daily headache syndrome, caused by the overuse (or abuse) of medication, usually analgesics. Analgesics remain an excellent and first-line medication for migraine. However, when they are used too frequently, especially for both tension-type headaches and migraine, they can become addictive. You can then get into a vicious circle of taking medication for a headache that is caused by the medication.

This syndrome should be considered as a cause of your headaches if they are occurring nearly every day and they are not responding to the usual migraine medications, as these will not work until the CDH has been eliminated. If you find that you are taking an increasing number of analgesics, you may need stronger medication rather than more of the same. You should consult your pharmacist or doctor.

However, if you do not have daily or near daily headaches, do not be worried that you might become addicted. This is highly unlikely if you keep to the amount recommended. Just keep it in mind if your headache frequency increases, but always consult your doctor to discuss it first, as there may be other reasons for an increased frequency of headaches.

Also, it is not always as simple as you might think to prevent CDH, as the major symptom of withdrawal from medication is severe headache, so you may need the help of a non-addictive pain-relieving medication. You may therefore need your doctor's help for withdrawal. Expect it to take at least ten days to two weeks to break this cycle of headaches.

Ergotamine, one of the drugs prescribed for migraine, and its derivatives can also cause this syndrome if overused.

CLUSTER HEADACHE

What is cluster headache?

In 1641, a famous Dutch physician, Nicolaas Tulp, who has since been immortalized in a painting by Rembrandt, gave the first convincing description of cluster headache and its typical cyclical pattern – an unbearable headache that comes at exactly the same time every day for 14 days (Koehler).

Cluster headache (also known as *migrainous neuralgia*) is, as the name implies, headaches that come in clusters, usually with freedom between clusters of months or years.

Its distinctive characteristics make it quite an easy condition to diagnose, yet as it is not a common form of headache, it is often overlooked by those unfamiliar with the condition and its symptoms. As with migraine, the cause of cluster headache is still unknown.

The symptoms

The headache itself can be the most excruciating of all headache disorders, often termed as being literally 'unbearable'. It is nearly always one-sided and occurs more on one side than the other. The most common site is orbital (around or to the side of the eye), next frontal (over the forehead) or temporal (at the temple) and then facial or dental.

Associated symptoms are a red, engorged, watery or running eye, nearly always on the same side (ipsilateral) as the headache (or occasionally both eyes are affected), nasal stuffiness, ptosis (where the eye droops) and miosis (where the pupil of the affected eye is constricted).

The phases

Kudrow (1993) has suggested that the best way of understanding cluster headache is to think of it as being composed of three major phases:

- the cluster phase
- the induction of attacks
- the attack phase.

The cluster phase

This is a self-limiting period when the sufferer is vulnerable and the 'window' in which the short, violent and frequent attacks can occur. This phase comes in cycles, as do the attacks themselves within the cluster phase. They are often reported as occurring at the same time of the year, peaking in January and July. This may be a response to the length of daylight or, more probably, the alteration in circadian rhythm as many attacks occur in the two weeks following the resetting of clocks backwards or forwards in summer and winter time and the sleep phase changes significantly at this time.

The induction of attacks

As with migraine, the cause of cluster headache is still unknown. We know from the symptoms that there are biochemical, hormonal and vascular changes, but data from the study of these is inconclusive. The internal carotid artery (the main artery supplying the brain, which is to be found at the side of the neck) and its offshoots are implicated, but it is not known for sure whether increase in blood flow in this region is the cause or result of the pain response. Some propositions put forward to explain this vulnerability are that it is a reaction to stress or an impairment of the central nervous system's response or its regulation.

Attacks are most likely to happen in periods of exertion, such as straining. Conversely, they may also happen in periods of relaxation, such as sleep, especially during the REM (rapid eye movement) period when dreams occur, usually in the small hours of the morning. They can also be triggered by high altitude.

Cluster headache can be provoked by vasodilators and histamines, although they only have this effect in the vulnerable cluster phase. It is also thought that it may be caused by hypoxemia – abnormally low concentrations of oxygen in the blood – over a long period. This may be why inhaling oxygen can abort an attack. Indeed, it is one of the major forms of treatment. It may be that the regulation of the blood's oxygen levels in cluster sufferers is faulty.

The attack phase

The attack phase, like the cluster or susceptibility phase, also goes in cycles. Headaches can occur between one and ten times a day. Sufferers who have only one attack daily are in the majority – 50 per cent – while another 25 per cent have two and the rest have attacks more frequently.

Attacks can be preceded by a time of euphoria, with yawning or a feeling of tiredness just before they start. They most commonly strike an hour or so after starting work in the morning. The next most common time is a few hours into sleep, the headaches often waking the sufferer in the very early hours of the morning. Whatever time they do occur, they are likely to follow the same pattern, occurring at the same time each day. The actual attack can last from only a few minutes or up to two or three hours.

An attack can start with a vague feeling of fullness in the head or neck or a feeling of warmth on one side of the forehead. Mild localized pain can then develop and intensify, with sharp stabbing sensations around the eye, temple or teeth on the affected side, with the pain finally coming to rest behind the affected eye. There is swelling, bringing pain in the temporal artery at the side of the forehead which can be partially relieved by pressing it with a finger.

With the developing pain comes a build-up of anxiety and fear of the pain that is to come. The patient may be liable to hyperventilate, pacing up and down as the pain builds. A pressure and force seems to grip the eye, boring and burning, with the pain growing in ever-increasing waves, subsiding slightly, then intensifying, again and again, until it reaches an excruciating level. This is sustained until the sufferer feels totally overwhelmed by the intensity of the pain, so much so that sometimes repeatedly banging their head on the wall in desperation as a counter pain is preferable to that of the headache.

At the height of the attack, clear fluid starts to stream from the eye.

As suddenly as they began, the waves of intensity start to subside to just being a severe pain, which, in comparison, is bearable to what has gone before. The sufferer then knows that they have again survived a pain they never thought they could.

How cluster headache differs from migraine

Migraine	Cluster
Family history of migraine usual	Family history of cluster unusual
Predominance female to male, 3:1	Predominance of male to female, 6:1
Aggravated by movement	Improved or unaffected by movement
Need to lie down	Cannot bear to lie down
Nausea and vomiting usual	Nausea and vomiting unusual
Younger average onset (20s to 30s)	Older average onset (40s to 50s)
Headache often of throbbing nature	Headache rarely of throbbing nature
Average frequency, 1 to 3 times a month	Average frequency, 1 to 3 times a day
Average length of attack. 1 day	Average length of attack. 1 hour
Propranolol is an excellent preventative drug	Propranolol has no effect
Lithium can make migraine worse	Lithium can make cluster better

The three major types

There are three major types of cluster headache.

- Episodic cluster headache *This is where there seem to be periods of susceptibility for the sufferer, with resistant periods of remission between the clusters.*
- Chronic cluster headache *With this type, there is no remission period, that is, the sufferer has a continuous susceptibility, but not necessarily continuous headaches. It can also be distinguished from the former type because it is particularly resistant to treatment. Proportionately, fewer women suffer this type.*
- Chronic paroxysmal hemicrania (CPH) *This type is thought to be a variant of cluster headache as it has many of the same symptoms, except that:*
  - individual attacks are shorter, but more frequent
  - it does not respond to the prophylactic medicines used for episodic and chronic cluster headache
  - it is easily treatable, as it responds extremely well to indomethacin, whereas episodic and chronic cluster headaches do not.

There are other types that should be mentioned, including cluster migraine – so-called as it has characteristics of both migraine and cluster headache. These can be either cluster symptoms occurring in a typical migraine attack (cluster migraine), or migrainous symptoms occurring during a cluster attack (migraine cluster). There is also a rare form of cluster vertigo, where episodes of vertigo occur during cluster headache attacks.

Who suffers from cluster?

Cluster headache is comparatively rare, so much less research has been done into the condition than that carried out into migraine. Of the world population, 1 in 100 suffers from cluster whereas 1 in 10 suffers migraine. However, as the condition has such distinctive symptoms, it can be identified much more easily than migraine, which makes research easier. One of the problems with migraine research is making sure that researchers are comparing like with like, that the same diagnostic criteria are being used.

As you have seen from the comparison of migraine and cluster above, cluster is mostly a condition suffered by males, usually the older male and only 1 in 100 of the general population suffer from it. John Graham, et al., noted that there is often a stereotypical cluster sufferer who is male, big and thickset, leathery skinned and liable to be a heavy drinker, but of course this is not necessarily the case.

Work recently done by Lee and David Kudrow has produced evidence to suggest that there is a genetic basis for cluster headache and also a genetic link between migraine and cluster headache, leading to the supposition that they may be the same condition.

Management of cluster headache

Your doctor is an important component in managing what can be a very frightening condition. Reassurance that there is no other underlying serious cause is important. Some doctors use substances to provoke an attack as a diagnostic tool and to watch the progress of an attack and try out treatments immediately. There are two or three substances that can nearly always provoke attacks in cluster sufferers. Diagnosis is not usually problematic.

It is useful to keep a diary of when your attacks occur and their frequency in any one cluster period. This is a good way of anticipating cluster periods and gives the doctor a good picture of your experience of attacks.

The best-known trigger of cluster headache is alcohol, but it is only a problem during the cluster cycle. In the remission period between clusters, it can be drunk without setting off an attack. It is therefore worth avoiding alcohol in the prone period. Nitrates and nitrites, which are added to such foods as meats to preserve them, should also be avoided. Diet does not seem to affect cluster headache as it does migraine. Some find relief in physical activity and pressing against the carotid artery at the side of the neck can also help.

The treatment of the acute attack of cluster

Oxygen therapy

Oxygen therapy, which was first used by B. T. Horton in 1956, has become a standard acute treatment for cluster headache, having been shown to be particularly effective in those who suffer from the episodic-type of cluster. It is thought to act by constricting distended cranial blood vessels.

The advantages of its use are that it:

- is extremely quick acting, with relief being experienced in as little as three minutes for some and seven on average
- produces a significant reduction of pain or aborts an attack if used early enough
- is safe, with no reported side-effects.

Most clinician's follow Kudrow's suggested treatment method, which is the inhalation of 100 per cent-oxygen at the rate of 7 litres per minute, using a loose-fitting face mask. When inhaling, it is important to sit upright or leaning forwards to achieve maximum benefit from it. Lying down while inhaling can actually aggravate rather than improve an attack.

The disadvantage is that:

• it is not always practical to use as you need quick access to an oxygen cylinder.

However, it can be used in hospital or a doctor's surgery, at the sufferer's home or place of work.

When the oxygen is taken is very important to its success. If you start using it at the very beginning of an attack, it is more likely to halt the progress of, or even abort, an attack. If you take it when the pain is at its most intense, it is likely to rapidly decrease the intensity. However, if you use it when the pain has got a significant grip, the pain is more likely to progress to its maximum intensity first, but from then on, relief can come quicker than would otherwise be the case (Igarashi, *et al.*).

Sumatriptan

The quickest acting form of sumatriptan, the auto-injector, has been shown to be the most effective pharmacological treatment for cluster. The response rate in trials was well above that for the placebo (an inert drug given to those taking part in the trial as if it were a real drug), the intensity of pain starting to decrease five to ten minutes after taking it. Do not take a second dose for the same attack.

Preventive treatment for cluster

For episodic cluster headache

Ergotamine

Ergotamine is used successfully as a preventive treatment for episodic cluster headache and has few side-effects. Treatment should be maintained for at least a month or until the cluster headache remits. It is sometimes used in acute attacks as well.

Merthysergide

This is a very effective treatment, but only as a preventive measure and is not as effective in chronic as in episodic cluster. Care has to be taken with administration and it should not be used for longer than three months at a time. This drug is more effective for younger sufferers (those under 35).

Pizotifen

Pizotifen is useful in prevention of both episodic and chronic cluster, especially where ergotamine cannot be used or is ineffective. Although pizotifen has been extensively used for migraine, over an extended period, not much is known of its use in cluster.

Verapamil

This is a widely used drug with few side-effects, but not much is written about it in the medical literature.

Lithium

Lithium carbonate is a good preventive treatment for cluster headache, especially chronic cluster headache. It is believed to act on nerve fibres. It has also been known to convert chronic cluster into an episodic type of cluster headache.

If you are prescribed lithium and the dose is high, you will be closely monitored while taking it and concentrations of lithium in the blood are monitored. This is because the dose may be close to the level at which unwanted side-effects occur. Some drugs cannot be taken while taking lithium.

For chronic cluster headache

All the following are used to treat chronic cluster:

- lithium
- verapamil
- pizotifen
- merthysergide.

Prognosis

You are less likely to grow out of cluster headache than migraine. Results of a study in Denmark by Krabbe that followed up 260 cluster headache sufferers concluded that, although less likely to grow out of their condition, they could develop longer remissions and that chronic cluster could change to the episodic type. In extremely severe chronic cases where all else has failed, surgery has been used with occasional success.

Migraine in childhood

My first encounter with children migraine sufferers is usually through a parent. If the parent is not a sufferer, or has had no close connection with migraine, then their reaction to the diagnosis of migraine in their child can be one of shock and so they are looking for information and reassurance. More often, the parent is a sufferer and knows only too well about the condition and how incapacitating it can be. They usually show a strong determination that their child will not suffer as they did. This could be a reaction to a general apathy on their part towards their own condition in that the average sufferer, when not having an attack, wants to forget about migraine or may feel that nothing more can be done in the management of their attacks. If only they had had the same attitude to their own attacks as they have to their child's.

HOW COMMON IS MIGRAINE IN CHILDREN?

Headache is a very common symptom in childhood and migraine is the most common cause of recurring headache. Migraine has been thought of as an adult condition only, probably reflecting extremely scant research into this subject until relatively recently. In the last 20 years, however, paediatric migraine has become recognized as a subspecialty. Special study groups and symposia on the subject now exist, together with a growing body of good and detailed research. However, very little information on this subject has been made accessible to parents and children until now. The only two books on the subject are both written primarily for clinicians and researchers (these are given in the Bibliography at the end of this book).

HOW MANY CHILDREN SUFFER?

The conclusions of migraine prevalence studies vary. The earliest was done in Scandinavia by Vahlquist in 1955 and looked at 10 to 12 year olds It showed that about 5 per cent of this age group suffer migraine attacks. Although quite a few studies have been carried out since then, with varying results, the most supported figure remains this one, that about 5 per cent of children suffer from migraine.

DIAGNOSIS

Diagnosis is always by means of the close evaluation of each individual case by a doctor, as the diagnosis of what causes a particular headache in a particular child can be problematic. It is rare for there to be no family history of migraine, but, even if there is, the pattern of symptoms manifesting in childhood migraine can differ from those in adults. This has led to the condition often going unrecognized and undiagnosed. Even now, migraine in childhood is underdiagnosed, either because the symptoms themselves are mild or because the symptoms are unusual when compared to those of the adult form. It is often only in retrospect, when many adults come to trace their migraine history to childhood symptoms, that their childhood migraine becomes apparent.

SPECIAL CHARACTERISTICS IN CHILDHOOD

Migraine attacks in childhood tend to be shorter and less severe than those in adults. The International Headache Society criteria for diagnosing headaches specifies migraine as strictly lasting 4 to 72 hours, but a supplement of the criteria has now indicated a 2-hour minimum in children. Even so, attacks can be of much shorter duration, sometimes lasting only half an hour. They usually occur with the same frequency as those of attacks in adults.

A typical attack

A child can be unusually exuberant in the morning, seeming perfectly healthy and full of energy. Suddenly they become quiet or start to yawn and become sluggish and irritable, saying they 'feel funny'. They might turn pale and start complaining of a tummy ache and feeling sick. They may be running a slight temperature and have a bit of a headache. They refuse lunch, saying they don't feel hungry so you take them to bed to lie down. After a couple of hours sleep, they are up and bouncing around as usual, feeling completely recovered. This scenario, which may sound all too familiar, may pass by unexplained, but could well be a typical childhood migraine attack.

The severity of the headache

From this example you will see that the most striking difference between a childhood migraine and most adult attacks is that the headache component of the attack is often not the major symptom, as it would be in an adult – indeed it is often the basis of most diagnoses of adult migraine. (If a headache *is* severe in a child, you should seek your doctor's advice.) The headache also tends to be less one-sided, sometimes extending over the front of the head or generalized with no particular focus, the tendency to favour a particular side developing at a later age. Headaches at the back of the head are rare in migraine.

Migraine variants are also more common among children and migraine syndromes can be experienced for years without headache or some other of the well-known migraine symptoms developing.

Abdominal symptoms

The major site affected in childhood migraine is usually the gastrointestinal tract, for example the stomach, giving rise to the term 'abdominal migraine', although some dislike this term, feeling it to be misleading. In fact, some doctors in the past would have ridiculed a diagnosis of abdominal migraine, thinking it a non-existent disorder. However, the symptoms are real enough and include stomach ache or pain, nausea and vomiting, loss of appetite and constipation or diarrhoea. Periodic attacks of unexplained (cyclical) vomiting in childhood may well be migrainous. Often they later develop into a more typical migrainous pattern. Periodic attacks of stomach ache that come and go throughout childhood and were blamed on something a child ate, even though the pain was not gripping, may have been migraine.

There can also be a tendency to suffer car or travel sickness and although this sickness is not caused by the migraine, it is often an indication that a child is prone to migraine when taken with other factors. Many adult sufferers have strong recollections of experiencing travel sickness as children. Indeed, half of all adult migraine sufferers experienced travel sickness when young.

Children can also experience giddiness and fever. Having visual aura is more unusual or not reported as often and, when present, does not last as long as it does in adults. Like adults, though, children can experience hypersensitivity to light. Mood changes are more common in childhood migraine than in the adult form.

Abdominal symptoms in adulthood

Adults can also suffer from abdominal migraine, although it is not very common. Usually, childhood sufferers' patterns just stay the same and do not progress into the adult form. This may be an advantage, according to your point of view. There is also a wider choice of drug treatments.

Treatment of the attack

If you suspect your child is starting a migraine attack, encourage them to eat something, even something light, as it may be low blood sugar levels that are triggering the attack. If they feel a little nauseous, try giving them a sugary drink. It is also quite valid to give a mild painkiller, such as paracetamol (aspirin is no longer recommended for children because of the worry of developing Reye's syndrome), to try and ward off an attack. Always make sure you give the dose recommended for your child's age. As in adults, the best form to take is the quicker acting soluble form. If they feel very nauseous, a suitable anti-emetic (a nausea suppressant) can be given about a quarter of an hour before the painkiller. Ask the doctor or pharmacist which would be suitable. Then get them to rest or sleep.

If your child's migraine is causing disruption to their life or they fear the attacks themselves, their doctor may try preventive medication under careful supervision. Make sure, however, that everything you can do to reduce the severity and incidence of attacks, such as identifying triggers, is done.

Non-drug treatments can also have their place. Labbe investigated how skin temperature biofeedback and autogenic training can reduce headache activity in children and what part practising the techniques at home can play. Her results showed that the treatment could decrease the frequency and duration of attacks and that children are more likely to stay symptom-free. These results confirm other research. Biofeedback is particularly good for children, perhaps because they can see the results happening before their eyes.

HOW TO HELP YOUR CHILD

Migraine can be genuinely distressing for children. It is important to try and involve the child with the condition as much as possible. Empowering is just as important in children as in adults.

Start with reassuring them about the condition and encourage them to take steps to manage it. You can give them as much information as their age will permit. Successful treatment will depend very much on their cooperation and, from their point of view, it is much easier for them to participate when they know about the condition, how it is triggered, what can make it worse, what can make it better, how it could be avoided, how to explain it to others, how to cope with an attack when it comes, how to learn to live with it. Point out how common migraine is and that there will probably be two or three other sufferers in their class or among their friends. In this way they will not feel so isolated. A great deal of the information on the management of migraine later on in this book can be used for children.

It is also important to talk to the school about your child's migraine and how they can best help to deal with it. Let your child's headteacher, form teacher and school nurse know what to do if an attack occurs during school time. Clear guidelines will ensure that disruption in the classroom is kept to a minimum. An attack can then be dealt with calmly, reassuringly and without fuss.

- Let them know how to recognize an attack as the warning signs are not always easy to identify, especially for someone outside the immediate family. If your child has distinctive symptoms, these could be explained.
- Explain that it may not always be necessary for your child to be sent home. Let them know that a short rest or sleep may often abort an attack, so lying down in a quiet, darkened room for an hour or so may be all that is needed.
- If your child takes medication for their attacks, discuss the feasibility of the school teacher or nurse administering this during an attack.

Parents and family circumstances can affect a child's attacks. It is natural to be concerned about a child with such a condition, but it is very easy for parents to become overprotective. The worst thing you can do is to make the child feel 'ill' or different to, or more delicate than, their friends. If *you* consider them to be delicate, they will come to think of *themselves* as being delicate. It is not helpful to a child to make them think of migraine as an excuse, especially as it need not be. Overprotected children are disadvantaged children.

Often all that is necessary is reassurance and advice. By all means be understanding, and do not trivialize the condition, but also be matter-of-fact and help your child to be so.

When a parent suffers from migraine, it is very easy for them to reinforce negative, unhelpful behaviour regarding pain in their children. This has been tested experimentally.

Children were asked to do a pain-inducing exercise in front of their mothers. Of the two groups tested, one group were chosen because they coped well with chronic pain, the other group because they did not. It was found that the non-coping children exhibited more negative behaviour during the exercises and had less encouragement from their mothers, some of whom even encouraged their children to give up. This would suggest that parents can, by their behaviour, cause their children to be less able to cope with pain than they could be.

HOW YOUR CHILD CAN HELP

Just as adults can achieve good management of their migraine attacks, so can children. We may think of children as not being able to participate in the management of their own condition or understand what is going on with their bodies or how to take care of themselves, but I think we tend to underestimate our children. It was thought that they could not accurately describe their own attacks, but this has been disproved. They can do so quite effectively.

You know best of all what your child will understand or what might be the best approach. For example, the most effective 'treatments' are to increase their food intake and make sure they do not skip meals. Lack of food and the resultant low blood sugar or, more accurately, the body's reaction to low blood sugar, is the single biggest trigger of migraine in children. Whatever treatment regime you follow, give your child enough details for it to make sense. Giving the reason behind an action is just as helpful for a child as it is for an adult.

We do not really know yet what causes migraine, so tell them this. They may grow up with a burning desire to find out what the causes are, which would be wonderful as we need more researchers! Obviously you will have to explain things in a way that is appropriate to the age of the child, but once you understand the problem, it is a small step to then translate the information into language that makes sense to them. Try asking them questions while you explain, to see if they understand.

Here are some of the things you can do to help your child avoid attacks.

- Teach them to recognize when an attack may be starting by watching our for any warning signs. If they get irritable for example, they may not realize that there is a link between this and their attacks. When they know what to look for, they can let you know when they occur and then you can take the appropriate steps to help.
- Tell them that we do not know what causes migraine, but that certain things may trigger attacks. Encourage them to take an active part in identifying these and avoiding triggers coinciding if possible. For example, if exercise and a certain food are found to be triggers, avoid exercising and then eating that food.
- If they are old enough, help them keep a diary to pinpoint triggers (see Daily diary sheet, page 158), but if they are too young to keep such a diary themselves, keep it for them.
- Tell them how important it is not to skip meals and or just have snacks, but to eat good foods with sufficient carbohydrates and nutrients. Stress how important it is to have a good breakfast before going to school.
- Point out that lack of sleep is a contributory factor in triggering many people's attacks. Watch out if an attack follows a late night.
- Anxiety and stress can also trigger attacks. Encourage your child to talk about what has been happening at school. This way, you can pick up on problems early on. If they are reluctant to go to school, this may indicate problems.

THE PROGNOSIS

Be reassured that childhood attacks tend to be less pronounced and are more likely to become less frequent, especially if they started having attacks at an early age. Also, a child's migraine can be managed well and effectively when the child knows as much as possible about their condition as they can feel more in control of it. And don't forget that as many as half of all children who have migraine become migraine-free adults.

4

THE MANAGEMENT OF MIGRAINE

Developing a strategy

TAKE A GOOD LOOK AT YOURSELF

Management starts with education – not only education about migraine and its treatment, but education about yourself. Up to this point you have learnt all about the condition, as though it were an object that you have been able to walk around, pick up and move about, so you could investigate it from every angle. Now it is time to look at yourself, because it is only when you know yourself that you can be effective in managing your migraine.

Blau and MacGregor (1995) studied the behaviour of migraine sufferers during attacks to test the hypothesis that their behaviour – retiring to bed, drawing the curtains, closing the door and a need to be alone, which a remarkably high proportion of the sufferers do – is the body's way of withdrawing from harmful stimuli, just like a person would automatically withdraw their hand from a flame. The study supported their hypothesis.

Do we instinctively respond in ways that will cure us, taking ourselves away from whatever is causing a problem, or is migraine itself a protective device as some believe? Whichever happens to be the case, there is no doubt that you can have a significant part to play in the management of your condition, whether your behaviour is automatic or considered.

STARTING FROM SCRATCH

Confirming the diagnosis

I suppose the first step is to start at the beginning and check that the diagnosis is correct. This may seem terribly basic, but it is worth doing as there is no point in going further in learning to manage and treat the wrong condition.

You must also make sure that there are no other conditions present, as this can significantly affect the success of your efforts. Any other conditions must be treated before tackling the migraine. For example, it is usual for migraine sufferers to have tension-type headaches between migraine attacks. If you do, you must learn to identify which headache is migraine and which is a tension-type headache as they can require different treatments. However, if you are having daily or near daily headaches, there is a possibility that you have developed a condition called chronic daily headache (CDH) as a result of the medications you take. This condition must also be cleared up as any medicines you take for migraine will not work if you are also suffering from CDH.

If your pattern of headaches has changed or your attacks are becoming more severe, you should go back to the doctor as a matter of course. If you are feeling particularly anxious or depressed, even though you directly relate this to having to live with the constant fear of a migraine attack, go to your doctor.

Reviewing your relationship with your doctor

Another basic necessity for success in migraine management is having a good working relationship with your doctor. Indeed many clinicians and researchers feel that this is key.

I emphasize the relationship aspect as I do not just mean that you need to have a good doctor. Nearly all doctors must be 'good' by definition. That is, they must have achieved a recognized standard in order to practice. Doctors, however, are also people and as such have different personalities. Some may be wonderful at putting you at your ease, some will be shy and say little. You may expect every doctor to fit your own picture of what they should be like. In the same way, doctors may make assumptions about their patients.

It may be that you already have an excellent relationship with your doctor. However, if you do not, see under How to get the most from your doctor, page 123, as it will help you appreciate the doctor's side of the relationship and how misunderstandings can occur. The relationship you have with your doctor is important as migraine is very much a long-term illness and it will be your local family doctor who will get to know you and support you over the years.

SELF-EMPOWERMENT

If you have been living with migraine for a long time, you will have many preconceived ideas. You may never even have thought that you *could* manage your condition. You may have accepted migraine passively, just responding to attacks as they come along and, when they become too painful, disrupting or frightening, going to the doctor for pills and handing over all responsibility for the condition to them. It may be that you have assumed there was nothing you could do.

The opposite is true – migraine is very much a condition that you *can* manage. The severity of attacks can be reduced and so can the length of attacks. You may even be able to abort attacks or prevent them happening at all if you can successfully identify and avoid triggers.

So, what sorts of things should you be re-examining?

- Have you ever tried to identify your trigger factors? Did you know that it is more unusual to have only *one* trigger factor? You are more likely to be prone to a combination of triggers that, when they come together, can put you over the threshold into an attack, but if they occur individually, they may not trigger attacks.

  If you haven't tried to identify your triggers, do you know how to? Do you know what to look for?

  Can you link attacks or worsening of attacks with life events? If your headaches became worse a year ago, did that coincide with a change in your job or house? Can you think of any circumstance that it could be attributable to? Did you change your perfume, your washing powder, get a cat, get married, join a club, a committee, experience a bereavement, go on a diet?

- Have you ever considered your lifestyle and how it could be impacting on your migraine? Could your lifestyle be contributing to attacks?
- Do you feel in charge of your life or does it seem to be in charge of you? Do you get enough relaxation, exercise, time to yourself, treats to look forward to? Are you organized or under pressure? Have you unrealistic expectations of yourself? Do you know how to say no?
- What drug treatments have you tried, for how long and what dosages did you try? List every one. Did you give each a proper trial? Did you stop taking any without telling the doctor (some people feel intimidated into accepting a

drug a doctor suggests, but as they do not feel confident in taking it, they don't)?

- If you accepted a drug, did you try it properly? If you are worried about it, ask the doctor questions, the answers to which will inform your decision. If you don't want to take it after this, say so. It is pointless taking it halfheartedly, perhaps taking smaller doses, missing doses or just stopping it after a couple of days or so because it does not work. List any drugs you feel you have not given a fair trial. (For more about drugs, see under Taking the medicine, page 115.)

EVALUATION

As you search for the best way to manage your migraine, you must have a proper baseline so you can compare and monitor your progress. It is no good guessing whether or not your attacks are improving – retrospective information is notoriously inaccurate. Even if improvements are slight, several slight improvements can make one quite significant improvement.

So, you need to evaluate improvements by comparing how you are now to how you were. It is therefore important to record how often you suffer, how long attacks last and how severe they are. Various tactics might improve one aspect, say how often you suffer, but may have no effect on severity or frequency. Keep a headache diary, noting all these aspects, and what treatments or medications you are taking and when. Keep the diary for at least six to eight attacks to allow you to have sufficient comparable information.

Prevention

Once you have started to identify trigger factors and your migraine attack threshold, you can try to prevent attacks happening by avoiding these triggers or making sure that triggers do not occur together. There may be some triggers that are impossible to avoid – high-pressure weather conditions for example – but you might be able to avoid other triggers when these weather conditions occur.

If a major trigger is stress, you must take steps to avoid it building up. It is easy to say, I know, but there is always room for improvement in your routines and there are many ways of dealing with it, which I will come to later on in this chapter.

Treatment

While you are seeking effective preventive measures, you will also be undergoing treatment of either a drug or non-drug kind to help contain or abort the attacks as they occur.

Evaluating treatment

Treatments should be evaluated. To do this you should know the basics about the treatment, so check the following with your doctor or relevant professional.

- What is the name of the drug and what sort of drug is it?
- What does the drug do?
- How soon should you expect to see results?
- How long should you try it?
- Can you take alcohol or other medication with it?
- What do you do if you miss a pill?
- Are you starting at the lowest dose?
- What side-effects are common?
- What should you do if they occur?

Write down their answers so you have a record of what they said that you can refer back to. I can remember when my children were small that the doctor gave me a small card to keep a record of all the vaccinations they were given with the dates.

Over the years, I needed to refer to those cards a surprising number of times because although I thought I would remember the information, I never did. What a good idea it would be to keep a similar record of the medications the doctor prescribes with their dosages and dates.

Evaluating the management

The more ways to prevent attacks that you find are successful, the less treatment you should need. Therefore you will need to evaluate the overall management at intervals to judge what your next steps should be.

Improvements in attacks could be due to the time of year, when some trigger is not present that is usually present at other times. If you keep accurate notes, you should be able to identify this. There is also the natural history of the condition to bear in mind. Improvements may be due to a natural improvement because of the 'lifecycle' of the condition, which would have occurred anyway (migraine tends to improve with age). The best way to check (if you want to chance it!) is to revert back to what you were doing before the treatment and see if this has any effect.

Keep an open mind. People tend to have two distinct approaches to treatment: drug or non-drug treatments, with the drug treatments usually being tried first and, when all have failed, non-drug treatments are turned to, possibly in desperation. With migraine you have more leeway than with many other conditions as treatments are not taken to cure, but to alleviate or prevent symptoms, so there is no harm in trying one particular treatment as opposed to another. You therefore have a wider choice. The only thing that will prevent you managing your migraine well is you.

Finding your trigger factors

WHAT ARE TRIGGER FACTORS?

As mentioned earlier, the mechanism that causes migraine is not yet understood, but we do know quite a lot about them. Most migraine attacks appear to be spontaneous, that is, they have no obvious precipitating factors. Although attacks have been artificially induced under clinical conditions by substances such as histamine or nitroglycerine, even in research using patients who have identified their trigger factors, only about half were able to induce attacks using these triggers. Thus evidence about triggers is rarely consistent and much of it is circumstantial.

This said, there are certain factors to which migraine sufferers are extremely sensitive and which can provoke migraine attacks. It is therefore worth taking the time to try and identify these factors.

When asked whether or not they know what triggers their attacks, a very high proportion of migraine sufferers I speak to, who do not know, invariably start citing a long list of foods they have looked at but no non-food factors are mentioned. Research shows that dietary factors are not as widely implicated as non-dietary ones, yet sufferers themselves consider food as one of the biggest, if not the only, cause of their attacks.

The fact is, anything can trigger an attack, *if a person is prone to that trigger*. It is important to keep this fact in mind when going through the process of trying to identify your own trigger factors. Remember that not all of your triggers may be mainstream ones (those that a large proportion of migraine sufferers are sensitive to) – it may be that you have a trigger very few other sufferers have.

IDENTIFYING YOUR TRIGGERS

Trying to identify this trigger or triggers can be quite compli-cated, but it is not an impossible task. You just need to under-stand how to approach the problem, be aware of the nature of these provoking factors and how to follow the clues you will come across. For example, you find that sometimes chocolate seems to trigger an attack, but sometimes you eat it and it has no effect. Is it or is it not a trigger and, if it is, why should it trigger an attack sometimes and not at other times?

First, just because you *usually* have an attack after eating *chocolate*, it does not necessarily mean that chocolate is one of your triggers. It may be that one of the first stages of your attack is a craving for sweet food and, as you love chocolate, you eat a bar. You then develop a full-blown migraine attack and you quite naturally assume that it is the chocolate that has caused the attack, when really it is the attack that is the cause of your eating chocolate. Also, it is a fact that anxiety can trig-ger a migraine attack. So, if you think chocolate is a trigger, the actual fear of an attack occurring after you have eaten chocolate could trigger one. As you can see, in these cases, chocolate is not a trigger, just an innocent bystander.

Let us now assume that chocolate *is* one of your triggers. Why is it that sometimes it triggers an attack and sometimes it does not? The answer is that it is unusual to have a single trig-ger – sufferers are usually sensitive to several triggers – so there is more to it than you might think. Imagine that every sufferer has a migraine attack threshold. If only a single trigger is present, you may still be below your threshold, but when this is combined with another trigger or triggers this may take you over your threshold into an attack.

For example, imagine you have three triggers, which hap-pen to be chocolate, high-pressure weather conditions and exercise. If you were to eat chocolate on a certain day, but the barometer reading was low and you had a lazy day at home relaxing, you may well not get an attack. However, if the air pressure is high, you run for the bus because you are late for work and then you eat a bar of chocolate, you will almost certainly have an attack. Thus, the presence of one or two triggers may mean that you are still under your threshold, but if all three occur close together, they may provoke an attack.

You can see from these examples that trying to find out whether or not something is a trigger is not that straightforward. It is important not to jump to conclusions before you have sufficient evidence and you must be aware of what is real evidence and what is not. As mentioned earlier, the process of tracking down your triggers can be extremely complicated, but the clues should be there – you have to play detective.

Trigger checklist
Do not forget that anything can be a trigger if you are prone to that trigger. However, below is a list of the kinds of triggers that are most often cited by sufferers, both anecdotally and as a result of research. This does not mean that you will be prone to all these triggers, but you may be prone to some or else you may not have a trigger on this list, but it will give you a general idea of just how varied these provoking factors can be.

These factors seem to fall naturally into three categories:

- external, environmental triggers, which originate outside the body, such as weather conditions
- internal factors, which originate inside the body (and could be called just the processes of being alive), such as hormonal changes or fatigue
- external triggers taken into our bodies, such as food that, perhaps because of our bodies' faulty processing of these substances, trigger attacks.

Let us look at each of these a little more closely.

External triggers

- These include environmental conditions, such as weather conditions, especially extremes of temperature, hot dry winds, low or high barometric pressure. Seasonal changes can also cause problems, with spring being a particularly bad time of the year for some.

- Looking at regular patterns can trigger an attack, like lines on a page (reading the regular lines on this page could be a problem if this trigger affects you), glaring sunlight or glare from a VDU screen. Good, *et al.*, have done some research into the use of rose-coloured glasses with children and have found such glasses to be effective in reducing the frequency of migraine attacks. With fluorescent lighting, it is thought that the flicker triggers attacks (try choosing ones with electronic starters when buying fluorescent lighting as this type does not flicker). Also prolonged viewing of the television can be a problem for some.

- Extremes of noise, both in volume or pitch – that is, loud or piercing sounds – can cause migraine.

- Intense smells, such as heavy scent or smoke, can also be triggers.

Internal triggers

- Hormonal changes – those occurring during the monthly menstrual cycle, especially at the start of menstruation and at ovulation – and at times of extended hormonal change, such as puberty, pregnancy and the menopause, can bring on an attack.

- Strong emotion and psychosocial stressors, including anxiety, depression, excitement, worry, shock and mental fatigue, can act as triggers.

- Physical fatigue, overexertion, lifting, bending, straining, even travel can cause problems, but if you are fit, you may be less liable to be affected. Get fit sensibly, though – see your doctor to work out a regime that is right for your circumstances.
- Lack of food, fasting, dieting, irregular meals – all can leave you open to an attack.
- High blood pressure.
- Another internal trigger can be lack of sleep or too much sleep, for example when you have a lie-in at the weekend.

Processing triggers
- Food can trigger attacks; the ones mostly mentioned as being a problem are fruit, especially citrus fruits, dairy products, cheese, especially the more mature kinds, chocolate, vegetables, seafood, fried or fatty foods, some tinned food and additives or those used to enhance taste or preservatives, such as those used in curing processes, drink, especially alcohol and then in particular red wine and sherry.
- Smoke and smoky atmospheres can be a trigger.
- Oral contraceptives can cause problems for some. If one type does not suit, try another.

Keeping a daily diary

It is best not to try and exclude foods one at a time, as this could take a great deal of time and, as mentioned earlier, it is more likely that there will be a combination of triggers, so avoiding one food will not necessarily identify it as a trigger.

It is better to keep a daily diary of everything you do (see Figure 1 on page 158). Include not only *what* you eat, but *when* you eat it, what the weather is like, what you do in the day, if you travel or take any exercise, what news you receive, for women, when menstruation occurs, what mood you are in and, of course, details of any migraine attack. Also, note the medications you use and when you take them. Look for absolutely anything that you think could be implicated in your attacks. Do not forget that anything could be a trigger for a person prone to that trigger. However, there is no point just excluding the best-known food triggers as these may not be triggers for you and you could just be impoverishing your diet for no reason.

Looking for a pattern

Keep this diary for about eight attacks. Use the diary sheet shown in Figure 1 on page 158, either photocopying it or laying a sheet of tracing paper over it and using it as a template. You can then look back at the 24 to 48 hours before each attack to see if a pattern emerges. There may be a group of things you have noted that seem to be present during the run up to each attack.

For example, say on five occasions there has been sunny weather, on four occasions you have overslept, you have eaten fish three times and there have been unusually hectic days prior to four attacks. You can see that although not exactly the same pattern is occurring before every attack, there is enough evidence to suggest that some or all of the items above are provoking factors for you. When enough of them combine, you are pushed over the threshold into an attack. For example, if stress, fatigue or strong emotion are causal factors for you, you may be able to find notes in your diary on other hectic days when no migraine attacks were in fact provoked, as this was the only trigger present. This would imply that it was not enough in itself to cause an attack.

If you find keeping a diary every day is just too tedious or time-consuming (in these circumstances you are unlikely to keep it up), you can try to keep a diary retrospectively. When you have a migraine attack, think back carefully over the 48 hours beforehand. This is unlikely to be as accurate as keeping the diary as you go along, but it can be helpful, especially if your case is relatively straightforward. Don't forget that all your triggers may not be evident at every attack. It is also possible that you are more sensitive to some triggers than to others.

When you cannot find a pattern

Although keeping a diary is a very successful way of finding out about precipitating factors, there are times when there is just no pattern at all to be found. You should then consider that whatever is triggering your attacks may be something that is present every day. One migraine sufferer's wife suddenly developed diabetes and had to give up sugar. To help and encourage her, he gave up sugar, too, and when he did his migraine disappeared. Sugar is added to so many foods and drinks that it would have been extremely difficult to track down this particular trigger otherwise.

When you suffer can be a clue

The time of day or the day of the week you have an attack can also be a clue as to the cause of that attack. If you suffer mostly at weekends, this could be for several reasons. You may be one of those people who tend to keep going at work on cups of tea or coffee, but drink relatively little of these drinks at weekends. In this case, you could be suffering from caffeine withdrawal, which is surprisingly common. This is relatively easy to overcome. You can either drink the same amount of tea or coffee at the weekends as you do during the week or try to cut down your caffeine intake slowly over several weeks (this is more difficult than you might think).

Alternatively, perhaps you always have a lie-in on Saturdays and Sundays. Too much sleep on these days could be triggering attacks or else it could be your body's reaction to low blood sugar, which has been brought about by breakfast being delayed by your lie-in. If you always have it on the same day of the week, it is highly likely that you have a regularly occurring trigger prior to attacks. For example, if you have attacks mostly on a Monday or Tuesday and you go walking every Sunday, suspect your walks.

A change of routine can also be problematic. See if sticking to a set routine brings improvements.

It is common to wake up with a migraine attack (mostly migraine without aura). However, because this is the case, research has been carried out to see if there is some provoking factor during the night that causes these early morning attacks. If it happens late morning, it could be caused by missing your breakfast.

The dental connection

As noted, it is common to wake with migraine, so researchers have looked at whether or not there might be something happening at night to cause or trigger attacks. The Migraine Trust funded a research project by J. G. Steele at Glasgow Dental School to fit occlusal splints (small plastic appliances) over the teeth of selected migraine sufferers at night as it was suspected that grinding one's teeth at night might be the cause of the migraine.

The findings showed that neither attacks of migraine with aura nor migraine without aura were reduced significantly by wearing the splints. However, it was found that there was a dramatic reduction in tension-type headache and, for two of those who took part, their almost daily headaches were eliminated.

Many migraine sufferers experience tension-type headaches between their migraine attacks and part of the strategy you will be developing is to identify these as separate entities (as they are often treated differently) and to make sure these are eliminated, as this will also have an effect on your migraine.

Stress and relaxation

Stress is a necessary and natural biological response – part of being alive. Its physiological, biochemical and clinical effects can be measured. If you are to achieve any goal, the stress response will maximize your energy and performance levels, be they physical or mental, inhibiting the biological processes that are not urgently needed and boosting the ones that are. When you go into that important meeting or interview, it will ensure you will be performing at your maximum potential.

What exactly happens to the body in this arousal period? The hypothalamus (a region of the front of the brain that controls several important functions of the body, such as body temperature, thirst and hunger) responds to a stimulus from one of the senses – perhaps a suspicious sound has been heard. This in turn causes the pituitary gland (at the base of the brain) to release various hormones, such as adrenaline or noradrenaline, chemical messengers that cause the sympathetic nervous system to make the body ready to run, fight or, in our modern world, deliver a performance to impress a client, for example. Extra oxygen is sent to the brain, so you can think quicker, and to the muscles, so you can react quicker, and energy reserves in the liver and the muscles are mobilized in the form of glucose to give you the wherewithall to react.

Good and bad stress

This extra energy was usually utilized when, many years ago, our ancestors confronted an enemy in a fight or fled to escape it and the body could then return to equilibrium after the danger has passed. But in the very different lifestyles of today, when the confrontation is more likely to be with your boss and there is no way you can either retaliate physically or run away, you just have to grin and bear it. Therefore the extra energy produced by the stress response is not utilized and if it is not dispersed, it is then that it can become counterproductive. Many migraine sufferers suspect that stress is a strong provoking factor in their attacks.

What are the signs?
How can you tell if you are stressed? Are you stressed at the moment?

- Is your forehead wrinkled up in a frown?
- Are your teeth clenched?
- Are your shoulders tensed?

Chances are that if you concentrate on your shoulders right now, you will be able to relax them further. Now tense your shoulders muscles up and hold them as tightly as you can for a couple of seconds. Now relax them slowly. This tensing and relaxing will have eliminated some of the stress in your shoulder muscles and often short exercises like this may be all you need. It is a simple technique that is just one of the ways in which you can rid yourself of stress. There are over 600 voluntary muscles in your body, which come in pairs. When overstress occurs, the heat and energy potential in them is converted into lactic acid and fatigue then occurs. Tensing and relaxing these muscles cause the lactic acid to be dispersed.

How to get rid of unwanted stress

You can do the above exercise wherever you are, even at your desk at work. There are other tactics that you can also use:

- get up and take a short break
- change the job you are doing at that moment, preferably to one that needs less concentration.
- try breathing deeply – breath in deeply and slowly, then breath out, emphasizing this exhalation, and repeat this movement several times.

If you feel you may benefit from such exercises, ask advice from your doctor or get a book about relaxation exercises (I give some suggestions about books and organizations that can help at the back of this book).

Self-expectation

Much has been said about a migraine personality. Certainly it has been noticed that many migraine sufferers are very conscientious people and set high goals for themselves, perhaps too high. If this is so in your case and you think stress is a contributory factor in your attacks, give serious thought to revising these goals to more realistic levels, supplanting them with ones that are more easily achievable. Learning to say no can also help prevent you overloading yourself. It is possible to say it politely – have a few good standard excuses ready so you do not offend – and it is essential if you are to reduce the stress of too much work or responsibility. Get others to help as well, by delegating.

Food

Putting the food trigger in perspective

There are many misconceptions about the importance of food as a trigger of migraine. As I mentioned earlier, it is curious that, although a wide variety of non-food triggers are known, the majority of sufferers I speak to cite only food triggers. When asked if they have tried to identify other triggers, many are surprised to learn just how many and how varied the non-food triggers that have been identified are.

This said, it is worth looking carefully at your food and drink intake, as long as you are aware that there are other triggers that you may also need to investigate. I cannot repeat it too often, anything can trigger an attack if you are prone to that trigger.

The food allergy connection

The term 'allergy' leads to a lot of misunderstanding. The medical profession uses the term only in its strictest sense, which is to refer to times when the body has a true allergic 'antigen-antibody' reaction to a substance taken into the body involving the immune system. These antigens provoke characteristic symptoms, producing specific immunoglobulin (IgE) antibodies specific to the allergic reaction, a reaction that can be detected. Asthma, for example, is a true allergic condition.

Unfortunately, allergies are not easy to identify. Allergy testing is notoriously inconclusive, many false positive or negative readings are produced. There are also many allergy clinics that are not regulated and may not be up to standard. Ask your doctor to recommend one if you wish to undergo tests.

Allergies themselves are even more common than migraine, so there are probably many individuals suffering from both conditions. However, in these people the allergy does not seem to be the cause of migraine. Equally, the symptoms of allergy, which can include headache, do not fulfill the criteria for migraine. Research carried out on migraine sufferers during and between migraine attacks found that the immune system does not seem to be involved for the majority of sufferers.

Allergic reaction or food intolerance?

When we say we are allergic to a particular food, do we mean that our immune system reacts in the way described above or do we mean we have what is clinically termed a 'food intolerance', which is a sensitivity to a particular food? It is more likely that we mean the latter. You can deal with this problem yourself, identifying the offending food by keeping a daily diary of your food intake during the 24 to 48 hours prior to a migraine attack.

You can also try an elimination diet, although these are much more difficult to keep to than you might think. Even subjects in trials, with tremendous support and direction, give up in large numbers. If you want to undertake one, go and get help from the doctor as your medical practice may have a nutritionist who could advise you. It is also wise to seek your doctor's help anyway as there is a chance that you will impoverish your diet if you eliminate foods without ensuring that you are still left with a nutritionally sound diet that will keep you healthy. Don't forget to keep a watch for non-dietary triggers at the same time. Read under Finding your trigger factors, page 69.

Additives

Preservatives, sweeteners, food colourings and flavour enhancers, E numbers – all have been blamed for triggering migraine attacks, but very little research has been done into this. However, although a bit difficult, it is not an insuperable task to go back to basics for a time. Cut these additives out of your diet by eating unprocessed foods – remember the potato? But don't forget that some meats and other seemingly basic foods are also processed, such as cured meats, fish and cheeses. Check the labels.

Not only what you eat but when you eat it – the role of low blood sugar

An enormous amount is said about diet being a trigger for migraine, yet probably of even more importance to the migraine sufferer is when you eat. It has long been recognized that going without food can make a sufferer susceptible to or even trigger an attack.

This link was first noticed in people who fasted as it was found that long periods without food could cause headaches of quite a severe nature, often accompanied by nausea. Also, the symptoms of going without food were surprisingly similar to the prodromes (early warning signs) of a migraine attack itself – yawning, going pale, mood changes and cravings for certain foods.

It is also significant that migraine is rare among diabetics, who have problems with the regulation of blood sugar. Indeed, when a migraine sufferer develops diabetes, their migraine usually disappears.

We all need energy to function, and we obtain this energy by consuming carbohydrates and converting these to forms of energy our bodies can use. One of these is glucose, which the blood then carries to wherever it is needed in the body. The brain is especially dependent on this glucose supply as it is virtually the brain's only fuel. When you eat, the levels of concentration of glucose in the blood – your blood sugar levels – go up. If the level of blood sugar goes too high this stimulates the release of the hormone insulin, which then brings the level down by removing some of this glucose from the blood and stimulating other cells, mostly in the liver or muscles, to store it for future use. When your body next needs energy, when the levels of blood sugar fall too low, the counterpart hormone to insulin, glucagon, is released. This stimulates the liver and muscle cells to release their stored energy and then the concentrations of blood sugar rise again. By means of this system we keep our blood-sugar levels regulated within a normal range.

Various problems can arise with our blood sugar regulation system. With illnesses such as diabetes, the body does not produce enough insulin and blood sugar concentrations get too high and when levels then drop too low, hypoglycaemia can result. However, symptoms of low blood sugar can occur even in healthy individuals, such as when you delay or miss a meal or you go on too strict a diet. Migraine sufferers seem to be particularly prone to the body's reaction to low blood sugar, especially children and people using large amounts of energy, like sportsmen and women. Deliberate fasting can produce a migraine attack.

It is not just a matter of consuming a snack with lots of calories to counteract the fasting either. If you didn't have time for breakfast, it is not enough to eat a chocolate bar mid-morning. The reason is that the sugars we consume in a normal meal are usually locked up in the foods we eat and are released slowly as our bodies break the food down. This ensures that neither of those upper or lower concentration levels are 'tripped'. When we eat a chocolate bar, however, we are consuming hundreds of instantly available calories, so, unless we use them immediately, they will quickly provoke blood sugar levels to rise dramatically, causing too much insulin to be released and this, in turn, will rapidly bring down blood sugar levels again, sometimes causing levels to drop too low. Also, we need the vitamins and minerals present in mealtime foods to metabolize sugar – there are very few of these in high-calorie snacks.

Some people who have a particular sensitivity to low blood sugar levels have found that having frequent small meals is better than two or three larger ones in the day.

Dieting and migraine

If you want to diet, take care not to do so too rapidly. There are several reasons for this. First, you will probably be more successful if you lose weight slowly as any weight you do lose is less likely to be put back on. It will also be easier to stick to the diet. Second, and of more significance to the management of your migraine, dieting too stringently can mean you will be going without food for long periods, which, as I mentioned, can cause your blood sugar levels to fall. If your attacks become more frequent during these fasting periods, bear this in mind and change your dieting strategy. You can still aim to lose the same amount of weight, but over a longer period of time.

Alcohol and caffeine

A number of research studies have been carried out regarding the possibility of alcohol precipitating attacks as many sufferers seem to be sensitive to alcohol. Complex alcohols and phenols, found in red wine, sherry and port, have been identified as the major culprits in triggering attacks. Further research is being done into why certain foods and drinks trigger attacks and the possible mechanisms involved.

The importance of a good diet

Diet plays an important part in generally maintaining good health and the ability to fight illness. A diet of good-quality foods in sufficient quantity is thus paramount for good health.

This is particularly good advice for migraine sufferers, whose hypersensitivity makes them prone to things that non-sufferers take in their stride.

Sleep

The role of sleep

The relationship between migraine and sleep is evident. We know that there is a definite relationship between them, but we do not know exactly what that relationship is. We only know that sleep and migraine share the same biophysiological mechanism as there is some evidence that the chemical messenger serotonin, which is involved in the mechanisms of a migraine attack, is also involved in the various stages of sleep. We know that migraine occurs during particular stages of sleep and can be affected by the amount of sleep you have – too little or too much sleep can trigger attacks.

The stages of sleep

Many attacks occur during or close to rapid eye movement (REM) sleep, which is when we dream and when increased autonomic activities (those functions the body carries out automatically) and resultant increased blood flow to the brain occur. Studies have suggested that migraine sufferers experience a high level of brain activity during this period and surges of noradrenaline have been found within the plasma of migraine subjects, this at a time when their levels should be falling.

Sleep as a treatment

Migraine has been treated by sleep rationing. As attacks also happen during deep sleep, waking migraine sufferers during this period was tried as a preventive treatment. However, this is certainly not a good idea for long-term treatment as sleep is so necessary for our general well-being.

Migraine can also be aborted by sleep, and it is often the case that a short sleep can be an almost magical way to achieve relief. Wilkinson, through treatment carried out at the City of London Migraine Clinic, confirmed this general wisdom and showed that even a rest during an attack was beneficial, but a sleep was best. Whenever this is an option for you, take advantage of it.

The menstrual cycle

The role of hormones

Many women recognize that their migraine is closely linked to their menstrual cycle. We have already looked at the role of hormones through the lifecycle and the changing effects it has on the pattern of migraine attacks (see page 28). Not much can be done to evade these effects, other than making sure that other triggers are avoided during those times of the cycle when you are particularly prone to attacks to reduce the odds of triggering an attack as much as possible.

Other cyclical phenomena

Patterns of migraine attacks can closely follow cyclical patterns, indicating that a link is present, even though we may not know what underlying biological processes are at work to explain why the links are there. We have seen links between migraine and sleep, migraine and the menstrual cycle and with circadian rhythms, especially in cluster headache. Studies looking at other endocrinological cycles are also being done and hopefully one day we *shall* know.

5

THE TREATMENTS

Developing a strategy

FINDING THE RIGHT TREATMENT

As descriptions of migraine have been with us since written records began, so have treatments. Ancient remedies included cauterization with a red hot poker (although it is not specified, I assume this was done to the head), popping garlic under the skin of the temple, tying baby alligators to the head, applying badger's brain to the affected area, even shaving the skull and applying a plaster poultice. The widespread cure-all of trepanning (boring a hole in the head) was also used in days gone by.

Fortunately, knowledge and treatments are now much improved and have become more scientifically based, guided by modern research techniques and findings. There is a wide variety of treatments, of the drug and non-drug kinds.

Comparing drug and non-drug forms of treatment

There is no getting away from the fact that many people dislike taking drugs. Indeed, some would go to any lengths and put up with a great deal of pain rather than take them. Others take the medication, but do so reluctantly, feeling they have no alternative in the face of the excruciating pain and variety of unpleasant symptoms their migraine can bring. They are uneasy about what the drug may be doing to their bodies, acutely aware that there may be unwanted side-effects or dangers if they exceed the stated dose. They are right to treat drugs with respect as no drug – from alcohol to those your doctor prescribes – is completely safe.

However, taking drugs reluctantly under these circumstances can lead to the very real problem of non-compliance – that is, when drugs are not taken properly. In this way, drugs that could be effective for patients are not only lost, but research findings on the assessment of these medications are distorted. This constitutes a serious problem for researchers and research is even being done into the problem of non-compliance itself, so serious is the problem perceived to be. Research done by Catarci, *et al.*, at the Princess Margaret Migraine Clinic in London used a special pill container that had an electronic event recorder in the lid so they could monitor when and how often the lid was removed to take a pill. The results showed that many patients were not taking the medications as directed and their conclusion was that the response rate of drugs (how successful they are) is closely linked with the compliance rate.

If you are trying a drug:

- make sure that you are taking it correctly by following the instructions exactly
- make sure you take it for long enough – some medicines take time to reach optimum potency
- read Taking the medicine, page 115.

Give the medication a fair chance or you may be losing out on a very effective one.

The reason drugs are tried as a first treatment is probably because there is nothing easier than taking a pill. It hardly needs any interaction from you, the patient, to be effective as long you take the right dose at the right time. The doctor's role is also relatively easy. They write out a prescription and hand it over, saying the magic words about how many to take a day and when, and the transaction is over. Also, most medications taken as directed will be safe and effective and doctors know this. There are time pressures on doctors – perhaps there is a full waiting room, home visits to do and so on.

There are effective non-drug treatments for migraine, too, and much research has been carried out to support this. The most straightforward and easiest to manage include relaxation techniques, biofeedback, stress management and cognitive therapy, plus mechanical methods, all of which I will discuss shortly.

However, to put these treatments into the context of the overall management of migraine, it is useful to point out a number of problems that arise when comparing these methods to conventional drug treatments. Though they are not very difficult to overcome, once you know what the problems are, they carry with them associated costs and availability implications, which may be why these types of treatment get overlooked. Do not forget that it need not be a matter of first trying conventional treatment (drugs) and then going on to alternative treatments if the drugs are ineffective. With migraine you are not taking drugs to *cure* the condition as there is no cure as yet – you are taking them to *manage* your migraine or *prevent* it happening. The order in which they are tried or whether or not you opt for a combination of the two is therefore not significant.

Non-drug treatments need commitment from the patient, and it is not at all easy to predict which particular method will suit which patient. Each individual will therefore need to spend quite some time liaising with their doctor or seeing a trained specialist to carry out these treatments or being trained and monitored in the various techniques, seeking help when coming up against problems, being given encouragement and reviewing the success of the outcomes experienced. This will cost time and resources, all which may be wasted if the patient is not fully committed to the treatment.

Quite a few alternative therapies, like homoeopathy and acupuncture, are available on the National Health Service.

Coping with an acute attack

One of the problems with a migraine attack is that when it is full blown, your digestion slows down dramatically and, any medication you take will not be absorbed, so will not be effective. Therefore, the sooner you take your medication the better. Also, as the body's response to pain is increased blood flow to the affected area, this can make the migraine worse.

Many sufferers have warnings of an impending attack. They may feel hungry or tired or elated or uneasy or any other of a wide variety of symptoms, which are usually particular to the sufferer. Environmental triggers are definitely a problem for some, and the incidence of triggers attributable to the work environment are high. You may be at your workplace for a large portion of the week so stresses and strains of such surroundings can also take their toll.

Research has been done to find out whether or not there are particular jobs or job areas that are that are more likely to provoke migraine than others. Marshall and Kessell did a survey in 1982 and it showed that non-manual workers suffered twice as much from migraine as manual workers. Could this be because of the stress levels involved or other factors, such as working with VDU screens?

Strategies to use at work

What do you do when you have an attack at work? It may not always be possible or advisable to go home and, indeed, it may not be necessary if you can abort or minimize the effects of an attack. Some ideas and techniques follow that may help you. Again, though, as migraine is so individual, there are no hard and fast rules. Some of them might sound contradictory, but these are all strategies that various sufferers have tried and found successful for them, so is worth trying them to see which work for you.

Carrying your medication with you

Always carry a supply of your own medication with you. As mentioned above, when a migraine strikes, the stomach goes into stasis, that is to say that the digestive processes slow down dramatically and so anything in the stomach is not properly digested. That includes the medication you may have just taken. If it is not absorbed it will not work. That is why it is so important that you take your medication early on in an attack. Analgesics that have been dissolved first are assimilated much faster by the body, so always choose a soluble form whenever possible. Some people even take a small flask of water with them if they are going on a train journey or similar place where water will not be easily available.

Letting others know

Many people fear admitting to their bosses that they are migraine sufferers as they think it might jeopardize their jobs. Of the general population, 98 per cent have experienced headaches, with varying degrees of severity, but not many – unless they themselves are migraine sufferers – will be able to appreciate what an attack is like. They do not realize what a profound impact migraine can have on the biochemical, metabolic and neurophysiological systems of the body – in other words, that it is not just a headache. If they did, they would be much more likely to be sympathetic and less suspicious when you have time off for a 'headache'.

If colleagues know in advance what they can do to help when you have an attack, they will be able to give you this help when you need it. When they know what to expect, they can respond positively. People generally do not like to feel helpless, so if they know you have particular premonitory symptoms – perhaps you turn pale – they could even know before you that an attack is on its way.

VDUs, lighting and patterns

Glare can trigger an attack in some people. Fluorescent lighting can be a particular problem if it flickers. Make sure that the type used has electronic starters as these do not flicker.

There are good antiglare screens available for most sizes of VDU and fixing of one of these onto your VDU can be helpful if glare or flicker is a problem for you. Make sure you site your screen away from direct light, too, so reflection is kept to a minimum.

One problem that sometimes arises as you get older is that your ability to focus changes, so even if you wear one pair of glasses for reading and another for seeing long distance, you may still need a further pair when focusing mid-distance, which is typically the distance a computer screen is from your eyes. Straining to focus mid-distance could trigger attacks but, again, only in those who are prone to this trigger. Otherwise, if there is eyestrain, then tension-type headaches may occur.

Posture

Correct posture is important for anyone sitting at a desk or VDU screen for prolonged periods. However, it may be a particular problem for a migraine sufferer whose migraine is brought on by stressed back and neck muscles. An upright and supported position is preferable, with frequent breaks being taken to relieve the build-up of muscle tension.

In the UK, there are legal guidelines for minimum standards for workstations that your organization must adhere to and you should make yourself aware of what these are.

Enough carbohydrates and enough breaks

It is sensible to take regular breaks during a working day. When you get up and walk around, your body has a chance to relax. Stretching and relaxing muscles releases any build-up of lactic acid in those muscles, such as shrugging your shoulders. There are even simple relaxation exercises that you can do at your desk. Learn some and try them out. Even extra oxygen taken in during a short period of deep breathing can help relieve tension.

Also, remember to keep up your blood sugar levels by never skipping breakfast or lunch. Snacks mid-morning and mid-afternoon can also be helpful if low blood sugar and its effects trigger attacks. As I have mentioned, skipping meals is a well-known and quite common trigger.

What else to look for

Absolutely anything could cause problems. These are some things to watch for as they have brought on migraine in other sufferers:

• smells – a colleague wearing perfume, perhaps, or the cleaner's spray polish

- stress through negativity or antagonism in relationships
- heavy workload
- stress you can put yourself under if you are disorganized

In fact, anything in the environment that puts the body or mind under stress can act as a trigger. Look closely at your surroundings and routine with a really critical eye and experiment where you can. If you keep a daily diary as recommended earlier, you can look back after a time to see what effects certain changes have had.

Jobs that preclude migraine sufferers

There are hardly any jobs having migraine should preclude you from, except diving, where migraine symptoms can closely resemble decompression sickness, and being a pilot, where proneness to loss of consciousness, such as in basilar migraine, would have obvious implications. In fact, these two professions do screen for certain types of migraine before employment. Driving as an occupation, if you suffer from migraine with aura, and have no prior warning signs, could also affect your safety and the safety of other road users depending how much warning you get of an attack.

Non-drug treatments

Where do you start?

Non-drug treatments have been found to be particularly effective in the treatment of headaches and a wide variety is available, so you may well have many questions.

- Who is likely to benefit from these treatments?
- How do you choose which one would be the best for you?
- To whom do you go to obtain such treatments?

- How will you acquire the necessary motivation and skills needed for them to be successful?

It is assumed that you have already followed the advice in the previous chapters on management, have found and avoid triggers that affect your attacks wherever possible and have made suitable changes in your diet, routine and lifestyle.

Non-drug treatments are particularly appropriate for children and pregnant and nursing mothers, for obvious reasons. They are the first choice of those who dislike or distrust drugs. They can also work for those who can accept the self-responsibility and the self-discipline that are necessary for many of them to succeed. You can be healthily sceptical of such treatments and still achieve a positive outcome, but you must be motivated and prepared to give the treatment a fair chance.

It is much easier to take a pill, but there are many advantages to taking fewer drugs. You will probably need the support of drugs as well to deal with the acute attacks – at least at first, while you are getting to grips with a technique.

When conventional medicine fails, as it can, or there is a loss of confidence in doctors with little time for consultation, there is obvious room for effective alternative treatments. Many of the treatments are also non-invasive.

Alternative treatments are better known as complementary medicine or non-conventional therapies. They are defined as techniques that are not part of a medical school curriculum. Of these, the five most commonly used are:

- acupuncture
- chiropractic
- homoeopathy
- herbalism
- osteopathy.

These have developed what the British Medical Association call 'discrete clinical disciplines'. This means that each of these branches of complementary medicine have established training and good practice and therefore have the most potential to be used alongside conventional medicine.

With university chairs now being set up in complementary medicine, the British Medical Association publishing books on recommended practice, the US initiating working groups for its scientific testing and Germany spending 10 per cent of its national turnover for pharmaceuticals on herbal medicines, what is generally called complementary treatment seems, at last, to be coming in from the cold.

Whether treatments come under the heading of complementary, alternative or unorthodox medicine or therapy, they have suffered from the lack of rigorous scientific testing and regulation that has laid them open to sharp practice by unscrupulous practitioners. There is also much ignorance surrounding these techniques, even among doctors. Yet, in the USA, where it is a big and profitable business, more patients visit complementary therapists than family doctors.

Many of these unconventional treatments used in migraine therapy are still marginal, either because insufficient research has been carried out on them or the research that *has* been done is flawed either by faulty methods in the setting up of the research or, sometimes, due to imprecise diagnoses or the incorrect assessment of results. Because of this we are still unsure as to whether or not some of these treatments are really as efficacious as their proponents say or whether they are no more effective than a placebo. There needs to be much more rigorous assessment so they can either join the ranks of conventional therapy or be discarded (Edmeads, 1993).

Although much of the modern structures of primary health care are not set up for non-drug treatments, they are now becoming more widely available. This is not only due to the fact that many drug treatments fail, but also because of the growing weight of evidence confirming many of them as valid alternatives.

Lack of regulation also leads to anomalies. For example, a myth has grown up that all herbs and compounds sold over the counter are safe, yet often the reality is that we do not know. Anyone can go and get a drug from a healthfood shop which has unknown side-effects and has undergone none of the strict trials and tests that most conventional medicines have done.

Take feverfew, the aromatic chrysanthemum plant *Tanacetum parthenium*, as an example. Its leaves are often used as a 'natural' remedy for migraine and, indeed, they have been used over many, many years and found to be an effective treatment for migraine by many sufferers. However, feverfew is also a drug and can induce abortion, so it should not be taken in pregnancy or by those women who expect to become pregnant. Also, when buying feverfew pills from a shop, exactly how efficacious many brands are is questionable, as they come under no regulatory control, so you may miss out on what could be a good treatment because the brand you are taking is not as effective as another.

So, you see, matters are not as straightforward as they would first appear. It is time that complementary therapies were put to the same tests as orthodox ones. It is only then that we can judge whether or not they are effective and worth the time, money and faith we put in them.

The British Medical Association has suggested guidelines for tests for complementary therapies in its excellent book, *Complementary Medicine: New Approaches to Good Practice*. There are also several useful, practical books, tapes or classes. For more in-depth information about most of the techniques, contact the organizations mentioned at the end of this book.

Mechanical ways of relieving pain

Many of the following are useful techniques for alleviating pain during an acute attack.

Temperature and pressure

Ice packs have been used extensively to relieve aches and pains. The application of ice (cryotherapy) is a technique that has been reviewed by Robbins (1989). It was probably discovered empirically and was known to the ancient Greeks as a pain reliever. It was used as a form of anaesthetic in the Middle Ages as it numbed the pain in the affected area. It is thought to work as a muscle relaxant and, by reducing blood flow to the area where the ice is applied, the distended blood vessels, which cause the pain, are made to contract again.

On a practical note, a pack of frozen peas can make an effective ice pack (but don't eat them after freezing and refreezing!) or a frozen coolant bag, such as the kind used for picnic boxes, is even more efficient, although less pliable when frozen than the bag of frozen peas. It can also be used again and again without problem. Some sufferers have found that having a cold shower can relieve their headache.

Heat can also relieve pain, as nearly everyone who has used a hot water bottle to relieve a stomach ache or toothache can attest. You can try:

- keeping a hot water bottle on the aching part of the head or sometimes on the back of the neck and shoulders
- hot or cold showers (it tends to be either one or the other that will work)
- a soak in a hot bath
- heating the hands or feet in hot water.

Pressure can also be used to relieve headache.

- Simple pressure against the temple can bring a certain amount of relief. In a study of 63 patients by Drummond, *et al.*, over a third obtained partial to almost complete relief by maintaining constant pressure against the superficial temporal artery in front of the ear. A sixth found further relief by compressing the carotid artery of the neck on the same side as the headache. Pressure applied to this point helped half of those not helped by pressure on the temporal artery.
- A bandage tied around the head can be helpful, but it can also constrict the whole head. A headband has been developed by Vijayan (1993) that presses rubber discs against the painful area by means of a wide (4–5-cm/ 1½–2-in) elastic-type band right around the head, with Velcro fastening to ensure a correct fit.
- One device – Migra-lief – uses cooling, warming and pressure methods combined and has been employed by Lance (1988). It is a soft helmet that uses compartments to deliver cold (2 degrees Centigrade) to the temples and back of the neck, and warmth (41 degrees Centigrade) to the top of the head.

None of these methods can be said to bring more than partial or temporary relief, but they have a useful place in coping with an acute attack.

Manipulation

Manipulation techniques, such as osteopathy, chiropractic and massage, are useful. Osteopathy is a system of diagnosis and treatment using the musculo-skeletal system. The principle is to use gentle manipulation to restore and maintain the proper functioning of the bones and muscles. Chiropractic treats mus-culo-skeletal complaints via manipulation and massage with emphasis being placed on spinal X-rays for diagnosis. Research outside the chiropractic profession has been limited and it is difficult to carry out completely unbiased studies in this area. However, in one study where they compared chiropractic techniques to other 'non-chiropractic' types of manipulation, the improvement experienced was about the same. Care must be taken to go to a fully trained professional, as damage can be done with chiropractic techniques if the person does not fully understand what they are doing.

There is also simple massage and reflexology (the manipu-lation of the feet and hands) and shiatsu, meaning 'finger pressure', which is a Japanese form of massage using pressure points all over the body. These are straightforward methods that can be carried out by practitioners or the individual or a friend or family member when they have learnt the techniques.

Again, not much systematically collected data is available on the effectiveness of these techniques, but even in some areas of orthodox medicine data is also poor. Well-designed quality research is needed in many areas.

Psychological and behavioural treatments
Such treatments have been found to be particularly effective in treating migraine. When migraine is triggered in part by psy-chological factors, psychological treatments have been found to be particularly effective. If you do find these bring relief, it does not necessarily mean that your migraine was caused by stress. These are primarily preventive treatments that can be used to reduce pain or stop headaches starting. Treatments are very much tailored to the individual.

Relaxation and biofeedback

Relaxation techniques include progressive muscle relaxation techniques and the use of breathing exercises. These combined treatments can be at least as effective as conventional pharmaceutical treatment, especially where disability is not too pronounced. In trials between 30 and 80 per cent reduction in both the severity and frequency of headache activity has been achieved, especially where stress or muscle contraction is a trigger factor.

Biofeedback is a means of controlling functions of the body that were originally thought to be entirely automatic and therefore beyond conscious control. Using biofeedback and relaxation techniques in combination can be particularly helpful. Biofeedback is short for 'biological feedback' and it is called this because it uses instruments to give visual or auditory feedback that a patient can use in helping them control certain functions of the autonomic nervous system, such as heart rate, blood pressure or skin temperature. Its use as a therapy for migraine was first discovered by accident when it was found that a patient being monitored during a relaxation therapy session aborted her migraine attack by consciously increasing the temperature of her hand.

One particular biofeedback technique, that of hand warming, can be a simple and effective way of relieving headache. This is how you do it:

- tape a small surface thermometer to your hand (your dominant hand gives the best result)
- concentrate on increasing the blood flow to that hand, hence raising the skin temperature
- check that the temperature is increasing by watching the thermometer reading.

At first this technique may take quite a while to master, but the more you try it, the quicker it becomes and you can eventually increase hand heat without using the thermometer. The increase in blood flow to the hand is thought to decrease blood flow in the head and therefore lessens or aborts the head pain, thought to be caused by distended blood vessels. This technique is particularly useful for children, who find the process of changing temperature by the power of thought a fascinating experience and for whom minimum drug use is to be encouraged.

More sophisticated machines and feedback techniques, such as cephalic artery and muscle tension biofeedback, are available. Once the techniques are learnt, the use of machines can often be discontinued as the feedback component is no longer needed.

Cognitive or stress-coping therapy

This technique calls for identifying stressors and your individual reactions to them, then re-educating your thoughts and imagination regarding these stressful situations, setting realistic goals and developing stress-coping techniques to manage these situations. Assertiveness and distraction strategies are also involved. This therapy is also used in conjunction with relaxation techniques.

Assessing the efficacy of treatments

When you undergo any treatment, baseline data about your migraine is essential if you are to measure progress. Some treatments may work initially, but improvements may not be maintained. The improvement may be due to the treatment or the placebo effect (when you think it is going to work, it does) or even the natural history of migraine, as migraine can disappear without any intervention. In fact, the older you get, the more likely that it will improve or cease.

To properly evaluate any treatment – drug and non-drug – you should have a baseline measurement of your migraine attacks. You should know before you start:

- how often you suffer
- how long attacks last
- how severe attacks are
- what medications you take for any attack and the dosages.

To do this properly, it is advisable to keep a record of attacks over a period of months or about six to eight attacks before embarking on any new treatment

Carry on recording the same details during each treatment. You then have a fair comparison when you come to evaluate the treatment. Psychological and quality-of-life improvements should also be noted.

Cost and availability of treatments

Being able to predict who will benefit from these treatments is useful as they not only take up much time, but also need resourcing. McGrath and Sorbi have distinguished predictors to identify those who are most likely to benefit. These are as follows:

- those who have shorter histories of headache
- those who have a positive or open mind towards treatments
- well-motivated participants
- high-frequency but intermittent headache sufferers
- younger sufferers
- those who had no assertive skills.

Poor results were predicted in sufferers of depression or the highly strung as well as those who had other physical conditions alongside their migraine.

They also brought together various strategies to improve cost-effectiveness, including:

* using primary health care professionals under medical supervision to deliver treatments
* treating groups rather than individuals
* making treatments home-based, so, for example, the primary learning sessions could be supplemented by subsequent home treatment carried out by the individual, with manuals, audio tapes and someone to telephone if necessary and a minimum of face-to-face supervision.

All the above could be interchangeable according to needs.

Drug treatments

Where do drugs come from?

In the past, drugs were obtained from plants and animals and were consumed in their natural form. Nowadays most are made synthetically, but they have the same molecular make-up as the originals. In other words, they are often chemical copies of the naturally occurring drugs. There are a few exceptions where the natural form of the drug is still used, but the synthetic drug is usually considered to be safer, as they can be controlled more precisely. In the last 50 years, our knowledge of drugs has grown enormously.

The safety of drugs

No drug is completely safe. All carry risks, though some have more risks than others, especially if they are not used correctly.

It is always a matter of weighing the benefits against the drawbacks. Take alcohol, for example. We like it for the pleasant effects it has on our mood, but it can also affect our judgement, when driving for instance, which could lead to serious accident or death. It can also lead to physical illnesses and death when taken in excess, usually over an extended period. However, when we know how much we can take safety and when not to take it, we can make judgements that enable us to minimize the risks. The same is true of drugs you take therapeutically, which are termed medicines.

There is the Committee on the Safety of Medicines (CSM) which sets the standards for the testing of new medicines. The two main criteria set are not only that a medicine should be safe but also that it be medically beneficial. The drug has to undergo agreed rigorous trials and testing procedures set by governments, which can last over ten years.

Side-effects

A drug acts on a specific site or sites in the body. For example, you may be taking a drug to treat a symptom, say, the pain of a headache, and the target site to achieve this may be particular blood vessels in the head. However, that drug may also affect other sites, perhaps blood vessels elsewhere in the body, and so cause unwanted, sometimes adverse, reactions. Further, each person's response to a drug is very individual and may affect one person in a particular way but not have that effect in another person.

Side-effects are not necessarily that obvious, they can be subtle. You may feel more tired than usual or have a dry mouth; you may just not feel yourself. Every side-effect, large or small, should be reported back to the doctor as, not only might it be significant and indicate that you should discontinue that particular medication, but it is also necessary in order to build up a side-effects profile for that particular drug. This is a useful and necessary way to learn more about a drug's mechanisms and contraindications.

Pharmacological principles of treating migraine

The choice of drugs when treating migraine should *always* be made on an individual basis – there is no standard treatment. Consideration will be given to how frequent your attacks are, the severity not only of the headache, but also associated symptoms, what you have already tried and what impact migraine has on your life. Which drug is chosen must also follow an accurate diagnosis of migraine, as drugs that help relieve one sort of headache could actually aggravate another.

There is a wide variety of drugs used to treat migraine, many of which act on quite different mechanisms in the body. According to which mechanism causes your particular attacks, there should be a drug that will work appropriately. Some drugs cannot be used by migraine sufferers who have other contraindicated conditions and this must of course also be taken into account.

Attacks themselves can differ in intensity in the same individual and it may be that each one is also treated differently – one requiring a milder drug than the other. If there is nausea present, this would indicate that an anti-sickness medication (an anti-emetic) should be included. How the medication is taken can also be quite crucial for success, speed of absorption being important, especially for those drugs taken to combat an acute attack. So you see, there are many things to consider when deciding which drug is best for you.

Acute or preventive drugs?

Abortive treatment – that is, treatment used to deal with an attack as it happens – is often sufficient. However, when using preventive treatments, most people will still have to deal with individual migraine attacks, even though they may be less frequent or less severe, so you need to know about both types.

Drugs available for acute attacks range from analgesics to the latest serotonin agonists. The prophylactic drugs are ones you take daily to either prevent attacks occurring or substantially reduce their frequency and severity. Prophylactic drugs may be indicated if you suffer migraine attacks more frequently than once a month. It may also be that, when deciding between acute or prophylactic drugs, the doctor will consider how severely migraine affects your life. You may feel that you cannot deal with acute attacks even when they happen less frequently.

When you take your medication may also be significant. There are drugs not only developed specifically for migraine, but drugs produced for other conditions that, it has been found, also help migraine. Take the case of people suffering from high blood pressure. Some who were given beta-blockers to bring down their blood pressure found that these drugs also greatly improved their migraine, either reducing the number or severity of their attacks or both and, in some cases, preventing attacks altogether. Also, some found that they took the drug for some months with no attacks and this beneficial effect carried on even after they had stopped taking the drug. Trials were initiated, testing beta-blockers against the usual migraine medications and against a placebo and the beta-blockers were found to be a good prophylactic treatment for migraine – all by chance. This has also been the case for other drugs, for migraine and other conditions.

In my discussions about various drugs in the following pages, I use their generic names rather than their brand names as I think these will be the most useful for you to know and remember, especially with analgesic drugs, which make up the major group of drugs effective for the majority of migraine attacks. There are so many brand names, with so many different formulations that to name them all would be more confusing than it would be helpful. The three major analgesics in use are aspirin, paracetamol and ibuprofen, and various additional drugs are combined with these, such as codeine or caffeine, according to the brand name, to improve their effectiveness.

Brand names also vary from country to country, lending further confusion. Thus, if you are in the UK and you are taking Sanomigran, in the US this is called Sandomigran. You can usually identify brand names as they always start with a capital letter, whereas generic names do not. They may also have a trademark symbol next to the name, usually the letters 'TM' printed small. However, whatever the brand name, the generic name must always be given by law, so you can check the exact generic drug content of any medication you are taking. Knowing this can help you save money as the same ingredients of a branded name analgesics can often be bought in their cheaper non-branded forms. Ask your pharmacist for advice.

Always, always read the box and any instructions that come with any medications you take or follow your doctor's precise instructions. Don't assume you know how to take a drug because you have been taking similar ones for years – you may have been taking them *wrongly* for years. Also, take heed of any relevant warnings on the packet. There is usually a maximum daily dose as well as a maximum four-hourly dose. Drugs can be dangerous if not taken correctly.

Drugs used for acute attacks

Analgesics and anti-emetics

Although there is a wide range of drugs used for migraine, simple analgesics remain the mainstay for the majority of sufferers and these drugs should not be underestimated.

The City of London Migraine Clinic, a clinic in the UK treating the severest cases of migraine, recommend taking an analgesic combined with a mild anti-emetic, such as metoclopramide, domperidone or an antihistamine if there is nausea present. This is one of the most efficient treatments, especially if it is taken as early as possible in an attack. The anti-emetic can serve a dual purpose, aiding the absorption of the analgesics into the bloodstream as well as combatting nausea. Some also help promote gastric emptying. It is usually taken before the analgesic.

Analgesics include non-steroidal anti-inflammatory drugs (NSAIDs). These inhibit prostaglandin production, thus reducing pain and inflammation. Included in this category are aspirin (acetylsalicyclic acid), which is used for mild to moderate pain, although this is now not recommended for children under 12 because of the risk of a rare reaction termed Reye's syndrome (a rare brain and liver disorder in children). It should also be avoided in pregnancy and while breastfeeding and can cause heartburn or stomach pains. Some people are allergic to aspirin. If you feel restless, have blurred vision, stomach pains, vomiting or experience ringing in the ears after taking aspirin, seek immediate medical advice.

Paracetamol (acetaminophen) is another effective analgesic and is the drug of choice when aspirin is not an option. It is very similar to aspirin, but without the anti-inflammatory activity. Particular care should be taken to keep to recommended doses and *immediate* treatment should be sought if you overdose. Paracetamol can be bought in a form that includes an antidote to the drug so you cannot seriously overdose on it.

Ibuprofen has similar effects to aspirin, but should not be taken with aspirin and alcohol should also be avoided – it may cause stomach upset. Naproxen sodium and sodium diclofenac are also useful and can be used as a preventive treatment, as can aspirin. Check with your doctor about dosages, as prophylactic dosages are often lower than those recommended during an attack. Indeed, a very extensive trial was carried out on 22 thousand male American doctors, half of whom took low doses of aspirin daily, resulting in a 20 per cent reduction in migraine (Buring, *et al.*).

As I mentioned earlier, many of these painkillers are rendered more potent by combining them with other drugs, such as codeine – a mild opiate which also has analgesic properties – or caffeine or an antihistamine. Codeine or analgesics containing codeine can cause dependency, though, so always check what the recommended daily and weekly dosages are as well as hourly dosages to avoid this problem. Its long-term use can also cause constipation. Codeine can be useful, though, if diarrhoea is a feature of attacks.

One of the major reasons analgesics fail is that they are not taken early enough in an attack. The earlier these drugs are taken in a migraine attack the better because when the migraine attack has taken hold, they are not readily absorbed. Taking analgesics in effervescent form is particularly recommended because then they are absorbed more quickly. Even so, they should be taken before the headache starts or immediately at its onset. Better still, take them as soon as an attack is on the way, in the aura stage or even before, at the prodromal stage. Clearly, it is important that you be able to recognize your own individual prodromal symptoms and that you have quick access to your medication, so carry it with you at all times.

Sedatives

Benzodiazipines are relaxants and induce sleep, but care must be taken to avoid taking them habitually. Buclizine is both an anti-emetic and a sedative. Sedatives are not widely used in the treatment of migraine because of the danger of habituation.

Ergotamine preparations

Ergotamine is a stronger drug for use in more severe attacks. It works by constricting the cranial blood vessels.

It is more effective if taken at the onset of an attack (within the first hour or hour and a half), but use during the aura phase is controversial as the aura itself is thought to be caused by a restriction of blood vessels and so many feel that further constriction by means of this drug is unwise.

This can be a very effective drug and it has been used for over 60 years for migraine, but its use must be strictly controlled and reviewed at regular intervals. Overuse can also lead to worsening migraine attacks, background headache and problems with circulation, so take great care never to take more than indicated.

Sumatriptan

Sumatriptan is a newly developed class of drug which acts as a 5-HT agonist. Ergotamine does this, but sumatriptan acts more selectively.

It has been found to be a very effective drug and in trials has been shown to be effective for up to 75 per cent of migraine sufferers. It is quick-acting, becoming effective within minutes to an hour, often aborting attacks completely. It is effective even at later stages of a migraine attack, unlike other acute phase drugs. Thus, for those sufferers who have no advance warning of attack, this has been a major advance.

It is not used during the aura stage of migraine with aura

and should not be taken by children or those over 65, as it has not yet undergone trials with these groups, and if certain other conditions are present.

Drugs used to prevent attacks

If you suffer more severely and frequently from migraine attacks – say, two or more attacks monthly – and this starts to interfere with your life, prophylactic drug treatments may be indicated as well as drugs for acute attacks. Although they do not always completely eliminate attacks, they can help decrease their overall frequency and severity.

Beta-blockers

Since beta-blockers were discovered to be effective in migraine, these drugs have become one of the main and most successful prophylactic treatments. Smaller doses than those taken for blood pressure are usually sufficient.

There are five used for migraine:

- propranolol
- metoprolol
- nadolol
- atenolol
- timolol,

of which propranolol is by far the most frequently used and extensive research has been carried out on it.

Many people fail with these drugs because they give them up too soon. It usually takes a few weeks before the benefits are seen. If after this time there is still no improvement in your attacks, go back to your doctor as the dosage may have to be increased. As with all beta-blockers, you should not stop taking them abruptly. Always consult your doctor first.

Antiserotonergic drugs

Pizotifen is another mainstay of prophylactic treatment. It is an antihistamine but its exact mechanism is unknown. It is thought to help migraine by blocking chemicals that act on the blood vessels of the brain.

Its major disadvantage is that it can lead to weight gain. This could be a result of metabolic changes or because the appetite is stimulated. If this does become a problem, discuss it with your doctor.

It can also cause drowsiness, but this effect tends to lessen with time. Note that alcohol increases its sedative effect.

Do not stop taking this drug without consulting your doctor.

Calcium channel blockers

These drugs were originally developed to treat high blood pressure and irregular heartbeat, but they were then found to be useful for preventing migraine, too. Flunarizine, verapamil, nifedipine and dilitiazem have been shown to be effective.

Some of the side-effects can be constipation, tiredness, nausea, dizziness and non-migrainous headaches. In a small percentage of people, the side-effects make it necessary to stop taking these drugs.

When they do not cause such problems, they are particularly useful in preventing or improving prodromal and aura symptoms within a few weeks and headaches after a few months.

Tricyclic antidepressants

If your doctor gives you antidepressants for your migraine, it does not mean that they think you are depressed and that your migraine is 'all in the mind'. Antidepressants, like beta-blockers, were discovered as being useful for migraine because those who suffered depression who took them also found that their migraine improved. The drugs have since been developed for migraine as well. Amitriptyline and imipramine are both used in migraine prophylaxis, although the first is only used for severe and frequent migraine attacks because of its unwanted side-effects.

Side-effects can include constipation and weight gain.

Feverfew

Although there have been no long-term prospective studies into its toxicity, feverfew (the chrysanthemum plant *Tanacetum parthenium*) has been used for centuries to treat headache and scientific research in recent years has showed it to bring about a reduction in the frequency of attacks and nausea symptoms.

Active ingredients in commercial preparations of feverfew vary enormously. You might like to try growing the plant itself, eating two or three small leaves daily.

Feverfew should not be taken in pregnancy or by those who expect to become pregnant as it can cause spontaneous abortion.

Finding the right drug for you

There is no one drug that is effective against migraine. Each person needs individual treatment according to their own particular symptoms, the severity and frequency of their attacks and the impact migraine has on their life.

It was not known why some drugs worked for some and not for others, but drugs themselves have given us a clue. Different drugs work on different mechanisms in the body. The fact that one drug works for one individual and another drug for another, indicates that there are different mechanisms at work in migraine. Until now, there was no way of telling which was the mechanism responsible for any one individual's migraine, but this may soon be a thing of the past. Genetic research promises that there will soon be a test to identify these mechanisms and, therefore, identify which drug will be effective for the particular mechanism.

However, for the moment, with so many drugs available, it is still a matter of trying each one until you find which is the right one for you. This is not always as simple as it sounds. In fact, I suspect that it is the single most important barrier to successful migraine management. Repeatedly, sufferers who have sought help from The Migraine Trust have complained that their doctor is not interested. On questioning them more closely, however, a good proportion say the reason they think this is because their doctor just gives them one drug after another. They are obviously translating this as a lack of interest on the part of the doctor, not realizing that there are so many drugs and that the doctor is probably starting with the mildest drug and progressing to the medium and stronger ones in search of the one that will be effective for that person. If you do not know that this is the case, you can get very disheartened when you try drug after drug without success.

Taking the medicine
It is essential to know how to take and assess a drug yourself, to make sure you are giving each drug a proper trial. Your doctor can suggest which to try, but it is your responsibility to ensure you are taking it properly – you will understand why this is important when you have read this section.

Why drug treatments fail
It is extremely important that you understand your treatment. When a drug does not work, you should always go back to your doctor and say so. Better still, ask the doctor to explain the type and action of the drug to you, ask if they are starting you on the lowest dose. Also, ask how long you should take

the drug before expecting to see an improvement as the therapeutic effects of many drugs take time to build up and results
may not be seen for weeks, which is the case for drugs like
beta-blockers. You will therefore have to be prepared to give
each drug and dosage a sufficient trial period.

How long should you try a drug?

Propranolol can have a positive long-term effect. If taken over
a period of time, it may not only prevent migraine, but, when
the drug is stopped, the beneficial effect can still continue, the
migraine not returning. You can therefore see that if you took
this drug but stopped taking it prematurely, you would,
through no fault of your own, be losing a very valuable drug or
the best drug or only drug for you. You may, as a result, be
given a stronger drug when it is unnecessary.

Do not forget that if you are not aware that one drug needs
to be taken in such a way, you may be equally liable to fail with
other drugs, for exactly the same reasons. This can lead you
into a situation of desperation when you feel you have tried
everything.

Finding the right dosage

As I mentioned earlier, another consideration for the doctor
besides finding the right drug. They have to find out what the
optimum therapeutic dose of that drug is for you. This is
because the bioavailibility of drugs vary – that is, the amount
of the drug that becomes available due to your own particular
biological make-up.

Your doctor will start prescribing a given drug at the lowest
dose and, then, if there is no effect, a higher dosage can be
tried and so on until the lowest dose that is shown to be effective is found. If you decide to stop taking the drug because
it does not work without telling your doctor, you may be

scuppering your doctor's strategy to find the best drug for you, so talk to your doctor before giving up.

Hints on taking the medicine

Taking pills with water is always a good idea as it helps them go down easily. Also, if you take a pill just before a meal when there is not much food in your stomach, it will be more quickly absorbed than when your stomach is full of food. However, sometimes pills specify being taken with a meal, so read the instructions carefully first. If you have a choice of formulation, choose the soluble or effervescent version, if available, as this works more quickly, an important consideration in migraine, which inhibits digestion quite severely.

What to do if you miss a pill

When you are taking medicine on a daily basis to prevent or diminish attacks, you may sometimes forget to take a pill or take it late. Always ask your doctor what to do in this case or else read the instructions carefully as they may provide this information. Better still, make sure you get into a routine where they are taken at the proper times. For example, you could put them by your toothbrush, if you have to take them first thing in the morning. If you are taking them daily, the longer you take them, the more likely you are to lose track of whether or not that day's dose has been taken. If your pills do not come packaged in such a way that it is easy to see whether or not you have had your tablet each day, such as the helpful blister packs, you can buy seven-compartment containers cheaply at most pharmacists and count out your weekly allowance beforehand, which will give you a visual check.

Migraine in pregnancy

CHANGES IN PATTERNS OF ATTACK

First, the good news. For many women, pregnancy brings about a considerable reduction in the severity and frequency of their migraine attacks, especially in those women whose migraine is closely linked to their menstrual cycle. In pregnancy, 70 per cent of women's attacks become greatly improved or they become migraine-free in the remaining six months. The bad news is that, for a small minority, pregnancy can actually aggravate attacks, especially in the first three months, although even with the most severe attacks, there is no evidence that this will have any adverse effect on the pregnancy.

There can also be a change in the type of migraine experienced by women when they are pregnant. Occasionally, attacks can change from migraine without aura to migraine with aura. Some even experience their very first attack in pregnancy.

Improvements in the attacks experienced during pregnancy can mean that they temporarily worsen after delivery. This might be due to the sudden drop in hormone levels, as is the case in true menstrual migraine, or else changes in serotonin metabolism. Whatever the reason, attacks soon improve again.

What can the quarter of all women who continue to suffer attacks during pregnancy and those who may suffer even more severely do to manage their migraine, especially as pregnancy can be a time when you may be more prone to attacks than usual?

SHOULD YOU TAKE DRUGS?

It is usually during the first three months that the foetus is most at risk, which is the time when migraine may be the most problematical for the unlucky few. Silberstein (1993) reports on a large research project undertaken – the Perinatal Collaborative Project – which studied the effects of drugs on 50,000 pregnancies. It showed little or no abnormalities, despite the potential risk of various drugs. However, research in this whole area is very limited and the opinion of the medical profession is somewhat divided on the subject of drugs during pregnancy. Some say that no drugs are safe or that they should be severely restricted because of the risk to the unborn child. Even aspirin is not usually recommended as it has been shown to have distinct effects on the mother and foetus, especially in later pregnancy. Some say that one can be reasonably confident about the safety of paracetamol.

The question as to whether or not it is safe to take a drug while pregnant or breastfeeding should be a matter you discuss at length with your doctor. Talk about which drugs you really are best advised not to take and which are the least likely to cross the placenta and therefore have less potential to adversely effect the foetus. The benefits of the drug will need to be weighed against the potential risk to your baby.

If you do take a drug such as paracetamol, make sure you take it in the soluble form as it starts to act more quickly and is absorbed into the bloodstream faster. Take the medication with a small snack if you can (even a piece of dry toast is helpful) if you are too nauseous to eat anything else.

Caffeine is also a drug and can lead to problems, including low birth weight, but if it is consumed in moderate amounts there should be no problem. Don't forget that tea as well as coffee contains caffeine and so do cola and cocoa products in the form of sweets and drinks.

Pregnancy is not a time to turn to herbal remedies in the belief they will be safer as this is not necessarily the case. Feverfew is a drug, albeit a natural one. However, if it is taken during pregnancy, it can induce spontaneous abortion and was in fact used for this purpose in the past. You should therefore not use it if you are pregnant or expecting to become pregnant.

NON-DRUG STRATEGIES

As mentioned earlier, it is the first three months that are likely to be the greatest problem if you are one of the unlucky few whose migraine worsens during pregnancy. Knowing that the suffering will be limited to this period will sometimes help you get through it, but there are things you can do to minimize the risks of attack. If you know you cannot take your usual medication, you can take steps to avoid attacks as far as possible.

There will be extra demands on you at this time, both biologically and emotionally. You cannot, nor should you expect to, do as much while you are pregnant as when you were not, especially as this could adversely affect your migraine. It is important that you organize yourself as much as you can so you do not put too much stress on yourself. Try getting all the family to take responsibility for housework or jobs that need to be done. It is in everybody's interests to work as a team and, hopefully, everyone will pull together more after the baby arrives as well.

Sleep is a wonderful way for the body to repair itself. Make sure you have enough rest, especially now your body has so many more demands being made on it. If you become tired and are unable to rest or lie down, change the job you are doing to something less onerous or get someone to help you with your task

Relaxation techniques are a must if you are tense and feel under pressure. If you already have a child or children, it may not be possible for you to get the amount and type of rest you should have (see under Stress and relaxation, page 77, for some ideas on how to wind down). Massage also has a place in relaxation, and your partner can be a great help with this.

Mechanical methods of pain relief can also be used. Biofeedback can be a helpful alternative to drugs for pain relief. In fact, any of the techniques covered under Non-drug treatments on page 94 can be tried. Keeping to a set routine as far as possible helps, too. So, do not suddenly decide that you need to decorate the nursery — it could put you under unnecessary stress. Leave that until after the baby has been born.

Make sure you have regular, nutritionally sound meals. Eat little but often to ensure your blood sugar levels are kept up. This should also help reduce any nausea you may experience. In fact, take care of yourself generally. To recap, remember to stick to a regular routine, eat regular, nourishing meals, do not get overtired and get enough rest and sleep.

Be consoled by the thought that if your attacks have become more severe, migraine patterns usually revert to normal after the baby has been born.

BREASTFEEDING

You should be aware that a small amount of any drug you are taking will also be present in your breast milk. The concentration of a drug appearing in your breast milk is small, usually about 1 to 2 per cent. However, always ask yourself the following questions.

- Is the drug really necessary?
- Is it the safest drug I can use?

If it is, also consider drugs that are eliminated quickly by the body.

If you are having to take a powerful drug, consider asking

your doctor to monitor the baby's blood levels to check that the drug concentration in its blood are not too high.

If you need to take a drug while breastfeeding your baby, you can minimize the concentration of the drug in your breast milk by taking any medication immediately after giving a feed. The highest concentration of the drug will then occur directly after the feed and by the time the next feed is due, concentrations will have fallen to the lowest levels you can make them.

6

FINDING HELP

How to get the most from your doctor

THE ROLE OF YOUR DOCTOR IN THE SUCCESSFUL
MANAGEMENT OF YOUR MIGRAINE

Migraine is a condition that responds extremely well to
self-help. There is also a great deal of scope for self-help. In
fact, with proper management and occasional help from an
appropriate medication, the majority of sufferers can live relatively migraine-free lives. Not surprisingly, one of the most
important aspects of its management is undoubtedly a strong
doctor-patient relationship. As we saw earlier, this is widely
acknowledged by those in the medical profession.

There are also many advantages to being treated by your
doctor for an ongoing condition. First, they know or will be
able to get to know you, your family and medical history, your
personal circumstances, the community in which you live and
so on – all of which can have a bearing on how successfully
your condition is managed. They will also have an overview of
how it has been managed and which treatments have been
tried so far. They therefore know all they need to know to be
able to put the problem into its proper context.

The doctor-patient relationship

How many sufferers never visit their doctor or have given up on their doctor because they feel marginalized, patronized or that their condition is trivialized. Don't feel depressed about this as doctors themselves have problems. Dr Richard Smith, Editor of the *British Medical Journal*, talks of his own experiences: 'That's what I dislike most about doctors – the way they patronize you, [you are] made to feel grateful for any service at all'.

Doctors vary, as do patients. The best doctor I ever had gave me his home telephone number on the third visit. I never did need to telephone him, but I cannot tell you how much confidence this gave me and my family.

It is perhaps understandable that we learn to play a passive role in illness and towards the medical profession in our society. As most of us do not have great medical knowledge and because the terminology is not in everyday use, we tend not only to leave anything medical to the doctor, we also push all responsibility over to them as well. We also expect doctors to fulfill their role according to our preconceived ideas. We don't even expect them to be individuals just like us – articulate or shy, conceited or dedicated. We don't dare complain or praise them or let them know how things are working out.

In countries where health service provision is free to those who need it, such as the United Kingdom, patients may feel that they do not have the right to question a doctor. In countries where it is not, patients may feel they can, as a matter of course, demand 'value for money'. Both of these reactions are distortions.

A relationship is one that you have to work at from both sides. A lot is said about a *doctor's* 'bedside manner', but how much is said of the *patient's*. Surely the patient also some responsibility regarding the success of a consultation. Morale is said to be very low among those in the medical profession today, with doctor's saying that their patients expect too much, they have too much paperwork and many wanting to give up practising. It may therefore be your responsibility to encourage your doctor, discussing treatments, being advised about not demanding treatments, following instructions properly and giving positive as well as negative feedback.

Whose responsibility is your treatment?

It may be that your doctor does not attach much significance to your migraine, but that may be your fault. Have you let your doctor know just how much migraine affects you, your quality of life or your family? That it may have such repercussions is not always appreciated. For example, if you suffer twice a month, this may not sound too bad and, indeed, many people suffer this often and can cope adequately. However, if you suffer severely, feeling lethargic and anxious for over a day, the next day suffering the most severe of headaches and vomiting, which continues into the next day, and then take another couple of days to recover completely, this is eight days a month when you are either completely unable to carry out ordinary daily tasks or struggling hard to do so. If you are also unable to predict when attacks will come, it does not take much imagination to see that this can cause considerable disruption or make it difficult to hold down a job, let alone build a career. It also restricts your availability to people who may depend on you, makes plans for important occasions uncertain and so on. If you do not make this clear, the doctor cannot appreciate the impact migraine has on your life. It is your responsibility to let them know. There is nothing to be lost in reminding the doctor – after all they are treating you as a person as well as your condition.

PLANNING A FIRST VISIT

On the very first visit, you should anticipate needing a longer appointment than normal. As there is no test for migraine, the diagnosis your doctor will have to make will rest heavily on the various details you will give. You can either arrange a longer visit with the doctor's receptionist or you could take the last appointment of a surgery.

Because of the way the primary health care system is set up in the UK, even if you ask for a longer appointment, your consultation can be a race against time. This is why it is vital to plan what you want to say beforehand and know what the doctor is likely to ask you and why. In this way, not only will you be able to give an accurate picture of your attacks and their effect on your life, but you will have more time for a useful discussion about your needs and the management and treatment of your migraine.

If you are feeling ill at the time, this will not help. That is why it is also important to see the doctor at times between attacks, when you haven't a migraine. Here are some ideas to make sure that you build a good relationship with your doctor and also become a discerning medical consumer.

TAKING A HEADACHE HISTORY

As there is no test for migraine, the majority of diagnoses will be based on the description you give your doctor. If a sufficient number of your answers fulfill certain criteria, then the diagnosis is confirmed. Many patients may feel that they should undergo tests and that the doctor is not concerned enough if they do not do any or send them for some. However, tests are only necessary where the diagnosis is not clear cut or other symptoms cloud the issue.

Although you may be sure that it is migraine, your doctor will need to consider other symptoms that might indicate that other conditions besides migraine are causing your symptoms or that might be coexisting with migraine (this is termed comorbidity). If either of these is the case, the other condition must be treated before treatment for migraine will be successful. The answers you give to the doctor's questions will also indicate what treatment or management you might need (see below for examples of the sorts of questions you can expect to be asked).

If the pattern of your attacks has recently changed, tell your doctor how and when and if there were any circumstances that coincided with the worsening of attacks, such as a change of job, starting HRT, a bereavement — anything, in fact, that might be significant.

The questions your doctor will ask you

As your attacks may vary, think of an average attack or the most common sort of attack you have when you answer your doctor's questions. For example, if you *usually* have a throbbing headache, but *occasionally* have a constant, aching headache or if your headache *mostly* originates on the right-hand side, but *occasionally* starts on the left or has no focus at all, say so. Most sufferers have to describe their symptoms in these generalized terms as attacks vary not only from person to person, but from attack to attack.

Below are some examples of the sorts of questions you will be asked about various aspects of your migraine.

- Onset *When did your headaches first develop? How old were you?*
- Frequency of attacks *How often do they occur — daily, weekly, monthly, several times a year? Do they appear regularly or are they spasmodic? Do they occur, on average, every few months, but you go through periods when they happen weekly, for no reason you can think of?*

- *Associated symptoms* Do you get other symptoms besides headache – such as nausea, visual disturbances, dislike of light or sound, anxiety, sweating? (A lot of symptoms at the beginning of an attack may be gradual or mild, so you may not even notice them as part of the attack. Keep a record of a few attacks, from beginning to end, to identify all these features.)
- *Duration of attacks* How long do your attacks last? Minutes, hours, days, every day?
- *Precipitating factors* Are there any factors that seem to trigger attacks, such as exercise, eating something, missing a meal or sleeping late? What makes it worse – movement, light? What makes it better?
- *Severity* How severe is the pain – mild, moderate or severe?
- *Site* In which part of the head does your headache start – on one side, over the forehead, behind one eye, all over the head? Does the site change from attack to attack?
- *Type* What type of head pain do you experience – throbbing, pounding, splitting, stabbing, aching? Do you get different types of headache on different occasions?
- *Duration of headache* How long does the headache last – seconds, minutes, hours, days, weeks, constant?
- *Timing* Do the headaches happen at any particular time of day or day of the week?
- *Hereditary factors* Do any of your blood relatives suffer from migraine?

The doctor will also need to know how far you have got in the management and treatment of your migraine. Whether or not you have tried to identify trigger factors, looked at your lifestyle – in fact, all the things you have been reading about so far. Your doctor will want to know what medications have been tried. They will probably already have your notes, but the list of drugs and dosages there will not tell them how long or how rigorously you took these drugs. If you feel that you have not given any of them a fair chance, say so, as the doctor may decide to try one again. You should really keep your own record of all drugs as a matter of course. Also tell the doctor what other treatments you have tried, like biofeedback, acupuncture, homoeopathy, dental splints and so on.

It is important that you think about your answers to the questions and these other areas beforehand as many of these things are likely to have happened a while ago and you need time to recall them properly or ask your friends or family to clarify events about which you are uncertain.

Questions you should ask your doctor

There will probably be questions that you need to ask your doctor. Some will be in response to what the doctor says, so you cannot prepare these, but there will be ones that are important to ask, either to help you understand things or to implement your treatment successfully.

If your doctor suggests a medication, ask about it. How does the drug work? What type of drug is it? How long will it take to start having an effect? How long should you try it before coming back? What are the common side-effects? Are there any side-effects that you should report immediately if they occur? Is there anything you should avoid while taking it, like alcohol or other drugs or substances? Do you really need the medication, that is, could you try changes in lifestyle and avoidance of triggers or non-drug treatments instead?

You should also discuss general management of migraine and where the suggested treatment will fit in. Ask what happens if the drug doesn't work? What will happen next? Are you being started on the lowest dose? How do you cope with the acute attacks that may still happen if it is a preventive drug?

Should you try non-drug treatments and, if so, when? If the doctor thinks *you* are interested, *they* will be interested. If you have read Chapter 5, you should know exactly what questions to ask.

Misunderstandings that can arise

If you know where misunderstandings can occur, how to help the doctor, keep aggravation to the minimum and get your message across, you have a good chance of building a strong and proactive relationship. As I said earlier, migraine is an ongoing condition and you will need to call on your doctor over the years for help and support, so it is worth working hard to establish as good a relationship with them as possible.

You will recall that the single most common complaint I hear from sufferers is that they think their doctor is not interested in their condition because they just dish out different drugs every time they go to see them. They do not realize that there are so many drugs for migraine, working on different mechanisms of the body, that this is often exactly what a concerned doctor will *have* to do – try each one – until the right one and the right dosage is found for that particular patient.

Medical terminology can be another prime reason for misunderstandings. For example, you may judge your attacks to be due to an allergy, but your doctor knows that it is unlikely as a true allergic reaction is quite uncommon. You, however, may mean by this that you have a sensitivity to certain foods. You are both talking about the same reaction, but the word 'allergy' means different things to each of you (see under The allergy connection, page 80). Or it can work the other way round. The doctor calls something a nervous reaction, which means that it is to do with the nerves, but you think they are implying that you are neurotic. It is best, therefore to describe things simply so you are not talking at cross purposes.

Points of friction

Don't ramble and give unnecessary information. If the doctor asks you how long you have had the present headache, don't start saying, 'I think it started Friday night or was it Saturday morning. Oh it *was* Friday because I remember my sister-in-law came round and ...' Order your thoughts. Prepare a concise account beforehand.

WHEN YOUR DOCTOR WILL REFER YOU TO
A SPECIALIST

The vast majority can manage their condition with the help of their doctor. However, in a small minority of cases, it may be indicated that you should be referred to a neurologist or a migraine clinic. This will probably be for one of three reasons. It may be that:

- the doctor needs confirmation of the diagnosis
- your migraine is particularly intractable or disabling – it does not respond to the treatments available
- you feel it is appropriate, but you should discuss the reasons with your doctor as they may know of other treatments that have not yet been tried.

Most doctors can cope with most types of migraine and, as mentioned earlier, they are in the best situation to do so. You should not take up a clinic place unless you need it as this can prevent someone who really needs the place from attending. If you are wondering whether or not you need to attend a clinic, discuss it with your doctor first.

A CLEAN SHEET

Not all of us have the chance of a 'clean sheet' with a new doctor. If you have had a less than successful relationship with your current doctor, perhaps there are ways in which you could improve it and give the relationship a 'new start'.

Remember that your doctor can provide:

- diagnoses
- reassurance
- expertise
- up-to-date solutions for management and treatment
- long-term encouragement and guidance.

You can provide:

- accurate information about your medical history, the management of your condition to date and the treatments you have tried
- good and accurate feedback to your doctor
- proper implementation of your doctor's recommendations
- encouragement by taking an interest in ensuring that the relationship is a good one.

YOUR RIGHTS

Here are some facts you may not know.

- You have a right to see your records if they are computerized or written records made after October 1991, except where your doctor thinks this might be detrimental to your health or someone else can be identified through your seeing them.
- Your doctor is not obliged to see you without an appointment if it is not an emergency. If it is an emergency, you have a right to be seen by a doctor, but not necessarily your doctor.

WHAT TO DO IF YOU CANNOT GET ON WITH
YOUR DOCTOR

If all else fails and you remain extremely dissatisfied with your doctor, you have the right to change doctors, although doctors also have the right to refuse to register a patient or to take existing patients off their list. To ask about how to do this without jeopardizing your 'reputation' with the new doctor (if they find out you have requested a move), get in touch with your local Family Practitioner Committee or Family Health Service Authority. All doctors' practices should have a practice leaflet that you can obtain which will give you an idea of its services and specialties. You don't have to give a reason for changing doctors, but you will probably be asked.

Clinics – where, when and how

A migraine clinic is a centre that can provide specialist help with the diagnosis and treatment of migraine and also provides a focus for medical education and research. It is usually linked to the neurology department of a hospital and directed by a consultant neurologist or a doctor with particular interest and expertise in the subject. That the director has clinical expertise and experience in this area is more important than their original specialty at medical school (Clifford Rose and Lipton).

WHEN DO YOU NEED A CLINIC?

The weight of evidence suggests that migraine is best treated within the family doctor-patient relationship, for reasons that were covered in the previous chapter, and, indeed, the majority of migraine patients are successfully treated at this level.

However, the following are reasons for doctors thinking that it is appropriate to send you to a clinic for specialist help:

- there is doubt about the diagnosis of migraine
  - this may be due to problems such as the presence of non-specific symptoms
  - a rarer form of migraine is suspected, one that the doctor may not be familiar with
  - other headaches besides migraine are present, which complicates diagnosis
  - other conditions besides migraine may be present (comorbidity)
- you have not responded to treatments
- your headaches are getting worse.

The most common reason for referral to a clinic is the presence of rebound headache due to ergotamine or analgesic addiction, which means that you experience daily or near-daily headaches as well as your usual migraine attacks. Interestingly, Blau and MacGregor, working at the City of London Migraine Clinic, surveyed family physicians' and patients' reasons for being referred to the clinic and then compared these with their own findings. The most common reason for the physicians' referrals was failure of response to treatment, whereas the majority of patients identified the reason as being an increase in the frequency of attacks.

You always need a referral letter from your doctor to attend a clinic. This is standard procedure.

WHAT ARE THE ADVANTAGES OF A CLINIC?

The clinic is a valuable resource and has many advantages. As specialists here see more migraine patients, a wider range of types of headache and migraine and are likely to have a particular interest in migraine, they will have more expertise in diagnosing more difficult or unusual cases. They can also offer a wider range of therapies as they can usually call on interdisciplinary staff, such as neurologists, psychologists who can help with triggers or cognitive treatments, nurses who can help with education and will be the frontline in communication and dentists who can help with specialist splint therapy and physiotherapists.

WHAT ARE THE DISADVANTAGES?
There is widespread consensus that migraine can be best managed by nurturing a good family doctor-patient relationship. Your doctor is nearby and thus accessible, knows you well and can give you continuing support over the years through what may be a long-term condition. Another disadvantage of attending a clinic is that there are not many around and you may have to travel quite a distance.

WHERE TO GO
The Migraine Trust set up the first such clinic in the world 20 years ago to treat those suffering an acute attack. This was called the City Clinic, but is now called the Princess Margaret Migraine Clinic. The Trust now helps set up and fund clinics throughout the UK so, hopefully, the accessibility of clinics will continue to improve (there is a list of clinics at the back of this book).

HOW TO PREPARE – WHAT TO EXPECT
The first difference you will notice at a clinic is the amount of time that will be spent on the first consultation. It will be a much longer, more in-depth interview than you will have experienced with your doctor. You will probably also be given a physical examination.

If you have the problem of intractable migraine, this is your chance to finally sort your problems out, so it is worth preparing for your visit here too. Here are some of the things you can do to save time, time that could be much better spent in discussion about problems and possible treatments later on in the consultation and it will help the specialist in their diagnosis:

- a headache diary, showing the dates your migraine attacks occur, their intensity and duration (if applicable, include details of the menstrual cycle, otherwise, note details of any other headaches, such as tension-type headaches, happening between attacks)
- a list of other symptoms that occur during an attack
- a list of the medications you have tried, the doses and the length of time you took them
- a list of other treatments you have tried
- the impact migraine has on your life.

Put down anything you feel may assist the specialist, and put them more fully in the picture.

It is always easier to sit down quietly beforehand and gather together such information than to try and remember things during the consultation, when you are under pressure.

THE FOLLOW-UP

In the UK, clinics prefer to prescribe medications through your doctor, as hospitals are allowed to make only a limited number of prescriptions and it helps to keep their costs down. Clarify with the specialist if this will be the case and quote some 'what if' scenarios, such as:

- 'What if this treatment does not work?'
- 'What if I need to see you again or need to ask some questions?'

CLINICAL RESEARCH

The other side of a clinic's role is the research side because it has access to a steady flow of migraine patients.

You will always be able to choose whether or not you take part in research or clinical trials. It obviously helps accumulate useful, sometimes crucial evidence to put towards the bigger research picture, but you may or may not wish to take part. When clinical trials for drugs are going on, you can sometimes have a chance to try brand new drugs before they are actually on the market. If you are uneasy about taking part, you are not obliged to do so. You have the right to ask any questions that you feel are appropriate to allow you to make an informed decision.

Who else can help?

SELF-HELP GROUPS

Self help is a vital part of your management of migraine. Self-help groups are another matter. Whether they are useful or not is very much a subjective matter. Some people find that they are extremely helpful; some find that these group meetings are just not their sort of thing at all. However, even if you have never thought of yourself as a person who joins things or would benefit from such a group, try one first before making up your mind. Many have found these much more helpful than they had anticipated.

As one of the main concerns of many migraine sufferers is a feeling of isolation, self-help groups are tailor-made to remedy this. They can also be a valuable source of new ideas. They provide an opportunity to meet other sufferers and who better to truly sympathize with you than another sufferer? It can be a great morale booster. Many groups just meet socially for mutual support. Some are more ambitious and invite speakers to come along and talk on topics of interest regarding migraine management.

If there is no self-help group in your area, why not get together with another sufferer or two and set one up yourself. An excellent self-help book is given in the Further reading section at the back of this book.

ORGANIZATIONS THAT GIVE HELP

There are very few organizations who help and support migraine and migraine sufferers – the number of organizations worldwide is in single figures.

I make no apology for telling you about the one I know best, The Migraine Trust, as I have been with the Trust for many years and have been privileged to have watched, and been instrumental in, its development over those years. However, there is a complete list of other organizations in the Useful addresses list at the back of this book and it is worth contacting those that interest you for further details.

The Migraine Trust is active in every area of migraine. It:

- funds research grants and fellowships
- encourages research by providing international symposia and workshops
- encourages new researchers into the field of migraine by providing studentships
- works to improve diagnosis and treatments of migraine by setting up and funding migraine clinics and providing courses for doctors and other health professionals
- provides help and support for sufferers, through an extensive free literature service, regular newsletters and helpline
- provides authoritative medical advice to a variety of constituencies.

If you need accurate information, advice or a listening ear, there are few to compare.

The role of those closest to you

Living with migraine can put great stress on relationships. Because of the strong familial tendency there may be more than one sufferer in your immediate family and this may help, but how can those closest to you support you best and how can you make their lives easier?

There are no easy answers to this question, but I would suggest that the more those around you can participate in the prevention, management and treatment of your migraine the better. Sometimes this will take the form of simply leaving you to lie down in a quiet, dark room, sometimes it could be by sharing tasks and keeping stress to the minimum, but mostly it will be by making sure you enjoy life together to the maximum when you are migraine-free.

7

THE WAY AHEAD

Current research

WHAT IS BEING DONE?

Although migraine has been with us for thousands of years, until about 15 years ago, very little was known about it. The Migraine Trust was one of the first dedicated organizations set up to encourage and fund research by making grants and fellowships. However, with advances in techniques and technology, our knowledge regarding migraine is rapidly expanding.

The same is the case with drugs available for its treatment. We now understand more about pain pathways, the mechanisms involved in migraine, and the role of 5-HT (the chemical messenger serotonin), which is thought to be implicated in migraine. Drugs are becoming more sophisticated as they target these mechanisms more closely.

THE INTERNATIONAL SCENE

Migraine is now known to be a worldwide problem as more and more research covering a wide variety of communities and cultures show similar percentages of their populations suffering. It is therefore not surprising that research is expanding so rapidly.

At the last international symposium of the Migraine Trust, there were research submissions from over 50 different countries. However, the Trust's symposium is still the only research conference dedicated to migraine. The International Headache Society's conference had a full day on migraine for the first time in 1993. Interest in migraine is growing significantly.

However, the United Kingdom has barely 200 neurologists and it has been difficult to attract new, young researchers into the field. Migraine has long been perceived as being too difficult. It is also less hi-tech than heart disease, for example, and less emotive than life-threatening diseases. It is also less tangible; you can see a broken leg or test for a viral illness, but pain is a personal and invisible matter.

SCIENTIFIC AND CLINICAL RESEARCH

There are several types of research:

- the purely scientific, usually laboratory-based research, looking mostly at the molecular and cellular level that is usually carried out at hospitals and universities, where individuals follow their own interests regarding different aspects of migraine
- active research, carried out with sufferers themselves, looking at the extent of the problem or the lifecycle of attacks and the collection of individual information during attacks and even between attacks
- the clinical trials, where migraine patients try new drugs or compare the efficacy of a new drug with one that is presently already available – the steps are always slow (since the start of the 1990s, the genetics of migraine has been at the cutting edge of research, due to the discovery that familial hemiplegic migraine and cluster headache have a genetic basis).

Taking part in research

Most of the clinical research, as the term itself implies, goes on at a clinic under clinical conditions. If you are asked or would like to take part in trials, you would be welcome. These are going on constantly throughout the world. Of particular interest are people who suffer from the rarer forms of migraine as these cases are harder to find and have 'scarcity' value, such as familial hemiplegic migraine sufferers.

Quality of life

THE IMPACT OF MIGRAINE

There is no doubt that migraine can cause severe stress in the sufferer, placing a considerable burden on them. Migraine constitutes a distinct disability to many sufferers. Tschannen, *et al.*, looked at the disability sufferers perceived themselves to have as a result of having migraine, together with the feelings of depression and anger and the effects of these. Their results showed a definite relationship between depression and their perceptions of themselves as being disabled, with anger being strongly related to the depression. Therefore, sufferers not only feel disabled during migraine attacks, but life in between attacks can be significantly affected, too.

There are other unforeseen ways in which migraine can impact your life. It can cause fear of the next attack, feelings of frustration, worry about losing your job or of overstraining a relationship, even despair. 'It's like a life sentence' is how one sufferer put it.

FACTORS AFFECTING PERCEPTION

How you perceive your state of well-being is central to whether or not you regard yourself as having a good or bad quality of life. It is not something that is easy to measure, just as pain itself is difficult to measure in anything other than very general terms. Individuals vary in their ability to cope with illness, in terms of their own inner strength and the support they get from others. So trying to equate frequency and severity of attacks with quality of life measurements is problematic. Yet, researchers are beginning to recognize that it is a valid variable when judging the outcomes and effectiveness of treatments. Several quality of life questionnaires have been developed to try and legitimize this very subjective matter, to try and quantify it in a more scientific way.

Dahlöf suggested a three-cornered health-related quality of life assessment (HQL) that included a measurement of general well-being, but also of actual health (the assessment of the symptom aspect was subjective, but the biological signs could be measured) and, finally, a totally objective measurement of welfare, to include such variables as days visiting hospital, off work, missed social activities and income.

Solomon, *et al.*, developed the Medical Outcomes Study (MOS) using interview and questionnaire components that produced a good measure of quality of life.

Being able to assess your quality of life has different uses. It can be used to assess the overall efficacy of a treatment. It can be used to assess one drug against other, so that a judgement can be made, not only as to whether or not the drug works in the way it should, but what price the subject has to pay for its efficacy. This 'price' could be the time it takes to work on each occasion and overall (some take weeks), side-effects, reliability or otherwise, its ability to abort attacks and at what stage of the attack it can do so. A further use is that it can make people aware of how profound an impact migraine may have on the sufferer.

THE BELITTLING OF MIGRAINE

Sufferers tend to feel isolated by their migraine. People who do not suffer do not appreciate that it is not *just* a headache. Because of this, there is another aspect of quality of life that is often overlooked – the guilt: 'People think it's my fault, or that I am doing something wrong', commented a sufferer.

One of the problems is that migraine has no status. There is no medical test, so you cannot prove you have it. Also, nearly 99 per cent of people have headaches, so most people think they know what a headache is. What they do not appreciate is not only the intensity of the headache, but the other far-reaching effects – that it is 'a headache all over the body' – and the effects of symptoms like the nausea or vomiting and other changes in the gastrointestinal tract, mood swings, inability sometimes to speak, see or think properly, sometimes loss of use of the limbs or consciousness itself. Also they cannot appreciate what it is like to know that you have got to face a life of fear of such attacks themselves and of having to let people down, because you never know when it might strike. There also seems to be the underlying fear that, because of the intensity of the pain, this time it might be something more serious, such as a brain tumour.

Migraine sufferers can feel a great deal of guilt – guilt because they have to take time off work and colleagues have to cover for them. Also, they worry that others are thinking they are missing work for a trivial reason. This can be the same throughout their social relationships, at work, at home, in everyday life.

Worrying what others think is a very real factor that can impact on a sufferer's quality of life in most profound ways. It has been found that migraine sufferers have a greater reduction in their quality of life than sufferers of much more serious conditions such as diabetes and heart disease and more psychological stress than those with life-threatening diseases such as cancer. This may be hard to believe, until you bring the full effects of migraine into the equation.

The way ahead

NO NEED TO APOLOGIZE

There is no need to apologize for or feel guilty about having migraine. There is an enormous weight of research to indicate that it is just as real a disease as any other. As we have seen, with the genetic advances now being made, a test for migraine is on the horizon, which will help to revolutionize its status within the medical profession. With the discovery of a test will come the ability to accurately pinpoint the mechanism of your attacks and, hence, which treatment will be most effective. There will be no more having to try drug after drug in a process of trial and error in order to find which is right for you.

RAISING AWARENESS

Increasing awareness of migraine and its widespread biological effects also means an increasing status for sufferers, which is why I initiated Migraine Awareness Weeks at The Migraine Trust in 1992 and each year the response from the Media and from sufferers themselves increases.

THERE IS ALWAYS SOMETHING YOU CAN DO

If you have read this book, you are taking one of the most important steps towards successfully managing your attacks – educating yourself about migraine and what you can do about it. Never stop that process. Ensure that you keep up to date with every aspect of management. Develop a strong relationship with your doctor by making them aware of how migraine affects you, so your needs can be appreciated. In turn, make sure you understand and follow treatment advice that the doctor gives you and do not forget to give feedback – it should be a joint relationship.

Join an organization that can give you the continuing support you need, like The Migraine Trust, which has a worldwide membership. Make sure that you take control of your migraine and its management, not be controlled by it.

TAKING IT A DAY AT A TIME

The hidden dimension in achieving this end is, of course, time. You cannot expect to achieve ideal management of your migraine in a week or two. It is a matter of taking a step at a time and a day at a time – like learning to walk – but, with every step taken, it becomes a little easier, and you get a little nearer.

The biggest obstacle you have to overcome is yourself. As a migraine sufferer, it is highly likely that as soon as an attack is over, you want to push everything to do with migraine out of your mind. This is especially the case if you have suffered since childhood and know no other way of life than a life with migraine. You need to change this. Work towards good management of your migraine when you are most receptive and your mind is working at optimum levels, which is when you are migraine-free.

WHAT TO AIM FOR – EVALUATING YOUR PROGRESS

As you take each step, make sure you have some kind of benchmark that you can use to see whether or not you are improving. This will also encourage you on the journey. For example:

- keep a record not only of your attacks but of when they happen and how severe they are

- keep a daily diary to record factors that may be triggering your attacks
- don't forget that there are many types of triggers, not just dietary ones, and that they usually come in groups rather than singly
- try to order your life so the impact of migraine is kept to a minimum
- make sure that you look after yourself by keeping healthy
- keep to a good diet
- get sufficient sleep
- get enough exercise.

It all sounds so simple, but it will take time to achieve. Take your first step today.

BIBLIOGRAPHY

Adams, F., *The Extant Works of Aretaeus the Cappadocian* (The Sydenham Society, London, 1856)

Barlow, C. F., *Headache and Migraine in Children* (Spastics International Medical Publications, 1984)

Bille, B., 'Migraine in Schoolchildren', *Acta Paediatrica*, 51, Suppl. 136–87, 1962

Blau, J. N., 'Resolution of Migraine Attacks: Sleep and the Recovery Phase', *Journal of Neurology, Neurosurgery and Psychiatry*, 45, 1982

Blau, J. N. (Ed.), *Migraine: Clinical, Therapeutic, Conceptual and Research Aspects* (Chapman and Hall, 1987)

Blau, J. N., 'A Note on Migraine Posture During Attacks', *Headache*, *33*, 9, 501–2, 1993

Blau, J. N., and Drummond, M. F., *Migraine* (Office of Health Economics, 1991)

Blau, J. N., and MacGregor, E. A., 'Migraine Consultations: A Triangle of Viewpoints', *Headache*, *35*, 2, 104–6, 1995

Bousser, M. G., et al., 'Prevention of Menstrual Migraine by Percutaneous Oestradiol Treatment', in *Advances in Headache Research*, F. Clifford Rose (Ed.) (Libbey, 1987)

Bryan, C. P. (Trans. of H. Joachim), *Ancient Egyptian Medicine: The Papyrus Ebers* (Ares Publishing, 1930)

British Medical Association, *Complementary Medicine: New Approaches to Good Practice* (Oxford University Press, 1993)

Buring, J. E., Peto, R., and Hennekens, C. H., 'Low-dose aspirin for Migraine Prophylaxis', *Journal of the American Medical Association*, 264, 1711–13, 1990

Catarci, T., Whitmarsh, T. E., Hering, R., and Steiner, T. J., 'Compliance and Migraine Prophylaxis: A Serious Potential Pitfall', 9th Migraine Trust International Symposium Abstracts 1994

Clifford Rose, F., 'The Pathogenesis of Migraine', Presidential Address to the Section of Neurology of the Royal Society of Medicine, 1991

Clifford Rose, F. (Ed.), *New Advances in Headache Research*, Vol. 4 (Smith-Gordon Nishimura, 1994)

Clifford Rose, F. (Ed.), *Leeds Castle Workshop Proceedings* (Elsevier, 1996)

Clifford Rose, F., and Lipton, R. B., 'Special Management Problems in the Headaches: Headache Clinics', *The Headaches*, Oleson, J., Tfelt-Hansen, P., and Welch, K M. A.(Eds) (Raven Press, 1993)

Cull, R. E., Wells, N. E. J., and Miocevich, M. I., 'The economic cost of migraine', *British Journal of Medical Economics*, 2, 1992

Dahlöf, C., 'Assessment of Health-related Quality of Life in Migraine', *Cephalalgia*, 13, 1993

de Belleroche, J., Joseph, R., and d'Andrea, G., 'Platelets and Migraine', in *The Headaches*, Oleson, J., Tfelt-Hansen, P., and Welch, K M. A.(Eds) (Raven Press, 1993)

Drummond, P. D., and Lance, J. W., 'Extracranial Vascular Changes and the Source of Pain in Migraine Headaches', *Annals of Neurology*, 13, 32–7, 1983

Edmeads, J., *Headache* (Sandoz Canada Inc., 1992)

Edmeads, J., 'Unconventional Techniques' in *The Headaches*, Oleson, J., Tfelt-Hansen, P., and Welch, K M. A. (Eds) (Raven Press, 1993)

Edmeads, J., 'The Diagnosis and Treatment of Migraine: A Clinician's View', *European Neurology*, 34, Suppl. 2, 2–5, 1994

Edmeads, J., 'Differential Diagnosis of Headache', *Migraine Update: Issue 10 Professional Postgraduate Services*, 1991

Ekbom, K., 'Treatment of Cluster Headache in Europe', *Headache*, 1, 65–70

Ernst, E., 'From Magic to Medicine', *New Scientist*, 1994

Good, P. A., Taylor, R. H., and Mortimer, M. J., 'The Use of Tinted Glasses in Childhood Migraine', *Headache*, September, 1991

Graham, J. R., Rogado, A. Z., Rahman, M., and Gramer, I. V., 'Some Physical, Physiological and Psychological Characteristics of Patients with Cluster Headache' in *Background to Migraine: Third British Migraine Symposium*, Cochrane, A. L. (Ed.) (Heinemann, 1970)

Harris, J. R., *Medicine: The Legacy of Egypt* (Oxford University Press, 1988)

Horton, B. T., 'Histamine Cephalgia', *Lancet*, 72, 92, 1952

Igarashi, H., Sakai, F., and Tazaki, Y., 'The Mechanism by which Oxygen Interrupts Cluster Headache', *Cephalalgia*, 11, 1991

International Headache Society, Headache Classification Committee, 'Classification and Diagnostic Criteria for Headache Disorders, Cranial Neuralgia and Facial Pain', *Cephalalgia*, 8, Suppl. 7, 1–96, 1988

Joseph, R., and Clifford Rose, F., 'Cluster Headache', *Princess Margaret Migraine Clinic / The Migraine Trust Factsheet*, 1994

Joutel, A., et al., 'A Gene for Familial Hemiplegic Migraine Maps to Chromosome', *Nature Genetics*, 5, 1, 40–45

Koehler, P. J., 'Prevalence of Headache in Tulp's *Observationes Medicae* (1641) with a Description of Cluster Headache', *Cephalalgia*, 13, 5, 318–20, 1993

Krabbe, A., 'The Prognosis of Cluster Headache' in *New Advances in Headache Research*, Vol. 2, Clifford Rose, F. (Ed.) (Smith-Gordon Nishimura, 1991)

Kudrow, D. B., 'Association of Sustained Oxyhemoglobin Desaturation and Onset of Cluster Headache Attacks', *Headache*, 30, 474–80, 1990

Kudrow, L., *Cluster Headache: Mechanisms and Management* (Chapman and Hall, 1980)

Kudrow, L., 'Pathogenesis of Cluster Headache' in *Headache: Diagnosis and Treatment*, Tollison, C. D., and Kunkel, R. S. (Williams and Wilkins, 1993)

Kudrow, L., and Kudrow, D. B., 'Inheritance of Cluster Headache and its Possible Link to Migraine', *Headache*, 34, 7P, 400–7, 1994

Labbe, E. E., 'Treatment of Childhood Migraine with Skin Temperature, Biofeedback, Autogenic Training and Home Practice: A Component Analysis', *Advances in Migraine Research*, Vol. 4 (Smith-Gordon Nishimura, 1994)

Lance, J., *Headache: Understanding, Alleviation* (Charles Scribner's Sons, 1975)

Lance, L. W., 'The Controlled Application of Cold and Heat by a New Device (Migra-lief Apparatus) in the Treatment of Headache', *Headache*, 458–61, August 1988

Levi, R., Edman, G., Ekbom, K., and Waldenlind, E., 'Episodic Cluster Headache 1: Personality and Some Neuropsychological Characteristics in Male Patients', *Headache*, *32*, 3, 119–25, 1991

Lipton, R. B., Stewart, W. F., and von Korff, M., 'Global impact of Migraine' in *New Advances in Headache Research*, Vol. 4, Clifford Rose, F. (Ed.) (Smith-Gordon Nishimura, 1994)

Lockett, D. M. C., and Campbell, J. F., 'The Effects of Aerobic Exercise', *Headache*, *32*, 1, 50–3, 1992

MacGregor, E. A., 'Visiting a Migraine Clinic', *Migraine News No 61* (The Migraine Trust, 1992)

McGrath, P. J., and Sorbi, M. J., 'Psychological Treatments' in *The Headaches*, Oleson, J., Tfelt-Hansan, P., and Welch, K. M. A. (Eds) (Raven Press, 1993)

Marshall, M., and Kessel, R., 'Aspects of Migraine in Occupational and Social Medicine' *Arbeitsmed, Sozialmed, Praventiomed*, 17, 291–6, 1982

Olesen, J., Tfelt-Hansen, P., and Welch, K. M. A. (Eds), *The Headaches* (Raven Press, 1993)

Olesen, J., 'Migraine with Aura and its Subforms' in *The Headaches*, Oleson, J., Tfelt-Hansan, P., and Welch, K. M. A. (Eds) (Raven Press, 1993)

Ornstein, R., and Sobel, D., 'Assessment of Health-related Quality of Life in Migraine', *Cephalalgia*, *13*, 233–7, 1993

Osterhaus, J., et al., 'The Burden of Migraine', *News in Headache*, *2*, 3, 1992

Passchier, J., 'Quality of Life and Disability in Children with Migraine', *Megrim*, *7*, 4–7, April, 1992

Peroutka, S. J., *The Genetic Basis of Migraine: Leeds Castle Workshop Proceedings* (Elsevier, 1996)

Perugini, M., Balottin, U., Scarbello, E., Rossi, G., and Lanzi, G., 'A Study of the Relational Characteristics in the Family of the Migrainous Child and the Importance of Life Events' in *New Advances in Headache Research*, Vol.2, Clifford Rose, F. (Ed.) (Smith-Gordon Nishimura, 1991)

Robbins, L., 'Cryotherapy for Headache', *Headache*, 29,10, 1989

Robbins, L., 'Precipitating Factors in Migraine: A Retrospective Review of 494 Patients', *Headache*, 34, 4, 1994

Sacks, O., *Migraine* (University of California Press, 1992)

Silberstein, S. D., 'Headaches and Women: Treatment of the Pregnant and Lactating Migraineur', *Headache*, *33*, 10, 533–40, 1993

Silberstein, S. D., 'Tension-type and Chronic Daily Headache: 1994 MacDonald Critchley Lecture', Presentation at the 10th Migraine Trust International Symposium, London.

Smith, R., 'Doctor with a Patient's Outlook', *BMA News Review*, April, 1994

Soloman, G. D., Skobieranda, F. G., and Gragg, L. A., 'Quality of Life and Wellbeing of Headache Patients Measured by the Medical Outcomes Study Instrument', *Headache*, 33, 7, 351–8, July/August, 1993

Steele, J. G., 'Migraine and the Dental Connection: Just How Effective Are Occlusal Splints', *The Migraine Trust Factsheet 4*, 1994

Tollison, C. D., and Kunkel, R. S. (Eds), *Headache: Diagnosis and Treatment* (Williams & Wilkins, 1993)

Tschannen, T. A., Duckro, P. N., and Margolis, R. B., and Tomazic, T. J., 'The Relationship of Anger, Depression, and Perceived Disability Among Headache Patients', *Headache*, *32*, 10, 1992

Uknis, A., and Silberstein, S. D., 'Migraine and Pregnancy', *Headache*, 372–4, 31, 6, 1991

Vahlquist, B., 'Migraine in Children', *International Archives of Allergy*, 7, 348–52, 1955

Vijayan, N., 'Head Band for Migraine Relief', *Headache*, 33, 1, 1993

Wilkinson, M., 'Migraine Treatments: The British Perspective', *Headache*, September, 1994

Wolff, H. G., *Headache and Other Head Pain* (Oxford University Press, 1963)

FURTHER READING

This list starts with books that are ideal for the average sufferer who has a non-scientific background and progresses on to books that are increasingly technical as you go down the list.

If you find that some are out of print, which is especially likely for those towards the top of the list, you could try your local library.

Blau, J. N., *Understanding Headaches and Migraine* (Which? Consumer Guides, 1991)

Sacks, O., *Migraine* (University of California Press, 1992)

British Medical Association, *New Guide to Medicines and Drugs* (Dorling Kindersley, 1994)

British Medical Association, *Complementary Medicine: New Approaches to Good Practice* (Oxford University Press, 1993)

Barlow, C. F., *Headaches and Migraine in Childhood* (Spastics International Publications, Blackwell Scientific Publications, Oxford; J. B. Lippincott Co., Philadelphia, 1984)

Hockaday, J. M. Ed.), *Migraine in Childhood* (Butterworth, 1988)

Kudrow, L., *Cluster Headache: Mechanisms and Management* (Chapman and Hall, 1980)

MIGRAINE CLINICS IN THE UK

Royal Victoria Hospital
Grosvenor Road
Belfast BT12 6BA

Royal Surrey County Hospital
Egerton Road
Guildford
Surrey GU2 5XX

The City of London Migraine Clinic
22 Charterhouse Square
London EC1M 6DX

The Princess Margaret Migraine
    Clinic
Charing Cross Hospital
Fulham Palace Road
London W6 8RF

Withington Hospital
Department of Neurology
West Didsbury
Manchester M20 8LR

Royal Preston Hospital
Sharoe Green Lane
Preston
Lancashire PR2 4HT

Bootham Park Hospital
Bootham
York
North Yorkshire YO3 7BY

The Leicester Royal Infirmary
Department of Neurology
Leicester LEI 5WW

Department of Clincal Neurology
Ipswich Hospital
Heath Road
Ipswich IP4 5PD

USEFUL ADDRESSES

Helpful organizations in the UK
The Migraine Trust
45 Great Ormond Street
London WC1N 3HZ

British Migraine Association
178a High Road
Byfleet
Surrey KT14 7ED

Relaxation for Living
29 Burwood Park Road
Walton-on-Thames
Surrey KT12 5LH

Carers National Association
29 Chilworth Mews
London W2 3RG

Canada
The (Canadian) Migraine
   Foundation
120 Carlton Street
Suite 210
Toronto
Ontario M5A 4K2
Canada

America
American Council for Headache
   Education (ACHE)
875 Kings Highway
Suite 200
West Deptford NJ 08096
USA

National Headache Federation
428 W St James Place 2nd Floor
Chicago
IL60614–2750
USA

Australia
Migraine Society of Australia
PO Box 2504
Kent Town
South Australia 5071

Alternative therapies
Aetherius Society (Healing)
757 Fulham Road
London SW6 5UO

British Acupuncture Association
   and Register
34 Alderney Street
London SW1V 4EU

British Allergy Foundation
St Bartholomews Hospital
West Smithfield
London EC1A 1BE

British Holistic Medical Association
179 Gloucester Place
London NW1 6DX

British Homoeopathic Association
27a Devonshire Street,
London W1N 1RJ

British Hypnotherapy Association
1 Wytham Place
London W1H 5WL

Chiropractic Advancement
   Association (CAA)
PO Box 1492
Trowbridge
Wiltshire BA14 9YZ

Confederation of Healing
   Organisations
113 High Street
Berkhamstead
Hertfordshire HP4 2DJ

Confederation of Tape Information
   Services
Project Office
79 High Street
Tarporley
Cheshire CW6 0AB

General Council and Register of
   Naturopaths
6 Netherall Gardens
London NW3 5RR

Homoeopathic Society
2 Powis Place
Great Ormond Street
London WC1N 3HT

Institute for Complementary
   Medicine
PO Box 194
London SE16 1QZ

Natural Association of
   Homoeopathic Groups
11 Wingle Tye Road
Burgess Hill
West Sussex RH15 9HR

Organic Living Association
St Mary's Villa
Hanley
Swan
Worcester WR8 0EA

Pain Concern UK
PO Box 318
Canterbury
Kent CT4 5DP

Pain Society
225 Bedford Square
London WC1B 3RA

Register of Traditional Chinese
   Medicine (RTCM)
19 Trinity Road
London N2 8JJ

Shiatsu Society
c/o 5 Foxcote
Wokingham
Berkshire RG11 3PG

TRIGGER CHECK CHART: DAY   DATE

	6 am	7	8	9	10	11
Getting up & going to bed times						
Bowel movement						
Food						
Drink						
Social or work activities						
Travel or exercise						
Weather						
Mood stress levels etc						
Menstrual cycle						
Medication						
Migraine attacks and severity						
Other						

Figure 1 Example of a daily diary sheet

2	3	4	5	6	7	8	9	10	11	12 mid-night

1.1 Migraine without aura

1.2 Migraine with aura
- **1.2.1** Migraine with typical aura
- **1.2.2** Migraine with prolonged aura
- **1.2.3** Familial hemiplegic migraine
- **1.2.4** Basilar migraine
- **1.2.5** Migraine aura without headache
- **1.2.6** Migraine with acute onset aura

1.3 Ophthalmoplegic migraine

1.4 Retinal migraine

1.5 Childhood periodic syndromes that may be precursors to or associated with migraine
- **1.5.1** Benign paroxysmal vertigo of childhood
- **1.5.2** Alternating hemiplegia of childhood

1.6 Complications of migraine
- **1.6.1** Status migrainous
- **1.6.2** Migrainous infarction

1.7 Migrainous disorder not fulfilling above criteria

Figure 2 International Headache Society classification of migraine (1988)

INDEX